A Guide to Musculoskeletal Radiology

Narendra Singh Kushwaha
Mohammad Baqar Abbas

A Guide to Musculoskeletal Radiology

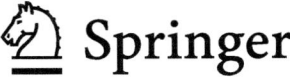 Springer

Narendra Singh Kushwaha
Department of Orthopedic Surgery
King George's Medical University
Lucknow, Uttar Pradesh, India

Mohammad Baqar Abbas
Department of Orthopedic Surgery
King George's Medical University
Lucknow, Uttar Pradesh, India

Department of Orthopaedic Surgery
Jawaharlal Nehru Medical College
Aligarh Muslim University
Aligarh, India

ISBN 978-981-99-6154-2   ISBN 978-981-99-6155-9   (eBook)
https://doi.org/10.1007/978-981-99-6155-9

This Springer imprint is published by the registered company Springer Nature Singapore Pte Ltd.
The registered company address is: 152 Beach Road, #21-01/04 Gateway East, Singapore 189721, Singapore

Paper in this product is recyclable.

Contents

Part I   Basics of Radiograph

1   Fundamentals of Reading a Radiograph   3
  1.1   General Considerations   3
  1.2   Conventional Radiography.   3
  1.3   Systematic Reading of X-Rays   4
  1.4   Rule of 2 in Radiography.   4
  1.5   Anatomy and Alignment   4
      1.5.1   Bone.   5
      1.5.2   Cartilage.   5
      1.5.3   Deformity and Density.   5
      1.5.4   Everything Else   5
  1.6   Radiographic Evaluation of Fractures   6
  1.7   Fracture Healing and Complications   8
  1.8   Radiographic Evaluation of Arthritides   9
  1.9   Radiographic Evaluation of Tumour and Tumour-Like Lesions   10
  1.10 Radiographic Evaluation of Musculoskeletal Infections   12
  1.11 Radiographic Evaluation of Metabolic and Endocrine Disorders . . .   14
  1.12 Shoulder.   15
  1.13 Cervical Spine (Fig. 1.12)   16
  1.14 The Acetabulum.   17
  1.15 The Ankle Joint   19
  1.16 Patella.   21
  Bibliography   22

Part II   Musculoskeletal Trauma

2   Radiographs of Upper Extremity: Fractures and Dislocations   25
  2.1   Shoulder Dislocation   25
  2.2   Scapula Fracture.   27
  2.3   Acromioclavicular Joint Disruption.   28
  2.4   Proximal Humerus Fractures   29
  2.5   Fracture Shaft Humerus.   31
  2.6   Intercondylar Humerus Fracture   32

2.7   Olecranon Fracture.   33
2.8   Elbow Dislocation   34
2.9   Radial Head Fracture   35
2.10   Monteggia Fracture Dislocation   36
2.11   Bado Classification   36
2.12   Galeazzi Fracture Dislocation   37
2.13   Distal Radius Fractures   38
2.14   Scaphoid Fracture   39
2.15   Metacarpal Fracture   40
Bibliography   41

3   **Radiographs of Lower Extremity: Fractures and Dislocations**   43
3.1   Hip Dislocation   43
3.2   Fracture Neck Femur   45
3.3   Intertrochanteric Fractures.   46
3.4   Subtrochanteric Fractures   47
3.5   Distal Femur Fractures.   48
3.6   Knee Dislocation   49
3.7   Patella Fracture   50
3.8   Proximal Tibia Fractures   51
3.9   Schatzker Classification.   51
3.10   Ankle Fractures   52
3.11   Talus Fracture.   54
3.12   Hawkins Classification of Talar Neck Fractures   54
3.13   Calcaneal Fractures   55
Bibliography   56

4   **Radiography of Spine Trauma**.   57
4.1   Cervical Spine Trauma.   57
4.2   Thoracolumbar Spine Trauma   58
Bibliography   59

5   **Radiographs of Pelvi-acetabular and Sacroiliac Region**   61
Bibliography   64

6   **Radiographs of Paediatric Orthopaedic Trauma**.   65
Bibliography   69

Part III   Orthopaedic Oncology

7   **Radiography in Orthopaedic Oncology**   73
7.1   Benign Primary Bone Tumours   74
7.1.1   Osteoid Osteoma   74
7.1.2   Giant Cell Tumour   75
7.1.3   Osteochondroma   75
7.1.4   Enchondroma.   76

      7.1.5   Chondroblastoma.. 77
      7.1.6   Fibrous Cortical Defect and Nonossifying Fibroma 78
      7.1.7   Fibrous Dysplasia....................................... 79
      7.1.8   Simple Bone Cyst 80
      7.1.9   Aneurysmal Bone Cyst 81
   Bibliography.. 82

8   Radiographs of Malignant Primary Bone Tumours 83
   8.1   Osteosarcoma... 83
   8.2   Chondrosarcoma 85
   8.3   Ewing Sarcoma 86
   8.4   Multiple Myeloma....................................... 87
   8.5   Adamantinoma.. 88
   Bibliography.. 89

9   Radiographs of Metastatic Bone Tumours...................... 91
   Bibliography.. 93

Part IV   Cold Orthopaedics

10   Radiographs of Upper Extremity Diseases...................... 97
   10.1   Osteoarthritis of Shoulder 97
   Bibliography.. 98

11   Radiographs of Lower Extremity Diseases...................... 99
   11.1   Osteoarthritis 99
   11.2   Osteoarthritis of Hip 99
   11.3   Osteoarthritis of Knee 100
   11.4   Osteoarthritis of Ankle................................. 101
   Bibliography... 102

12   Radiographs of Spine Region (Deformity) 103
   12.1   Scoliosis... 103
   Bibliography... 106

**13   Radiographs of Congenital and Developmental
      Skeletal Disorders**.. 107
   Bibliography... 115

Part V   Musculoskeletal Infections

14   Radiographs of Musculoskeletal Infections 119
   14.1   Pyogenic Osteomyelitis................................. 119
   14.2   Infectious Arthritis..................................... 122
   14.3   Tuberculosis of Spine.................................. 125
   Bibliography... 126

Part VI   Metabolic and Endocrine Skeletal Disorders

15   Radiographs of Metabolic and Endocrine Skeletal Disorders 129
        15.1   Osteoporosis. 130
        15.2   Rickets and Osteomalacia 130
        15.3   Hyperparathyroidism 133
        Bibliography 134

Part VII   Orthopaedic Surgical Procedures

16   Radiographs of Post-Surgical Orthopaedic Complications 137

17   Radiographs of Orthopaedic Reconstructive Procedures 149
        17.1   Fracture Fixation Implants. 149
        17.2   Joint Replacement Implants. 150

About the Authors

Narendra Singh Kushwaha, MBBS, MS, FICS, FSR, MNAMS post-graduated from M.L.N Medical College, Allahabad, India. He is a consultant orthopaedic surgeon (additional professor) at the Department of Orthopaedic Surgery, King George's Medical University, Lucknow, India. He has a special interest in the field of arthroplasty and arthroscopy. He has published many original research papers in various peer-reviewed international and national journals and has delivered numerous scientific oral and poster presentations at various international and national conferences. He was awarded APAS-Depuy synthes international fellowship in arthroplasty in 2022 (India, Malaysia, Australia, and Indonesia), IOA-Senior inland fellowship in 2021, IAA national fellowship in arthroplasty in 2019, AO trauma international fellowship in 2018 (Hong Kong), IOA-WOC national fellowship by the Indian Orthopedic Association in 2017, a fellowship of the International College of Surgeons (FICS) in 2014, and a fellowship in sport rehabilitation (FSR) by Medvarsity and Apollo Hospitals Educational and Research Foundation in 2014. He has been awarded with International Exemplary Research and Performance Award for excellence in orthopaedic surgery in 2018. He has been conferred several best papers and best poster awards at national and international conferences. He is a life member of various national and international academic bodies.

Mohammad Baqar Abbas, MBBS, MS post-graduated from J.N Medical College, AMU, Aligarh, India. He was a senior resident at the Department of Orthopaedic Surgery, King George's Medical University (KGMU), Lucknow, India. He has done his post-doctoral certificate course (PDCC) in arthroplasty at KGMU, Lucknow. Currently, he is working as an assistant professor at the Department of Orthopaedic Surgery, J.N Medical College, AMU, Aligarh, India.

Part I

Basics of Radiograph

Fundamentals of Reading a Radiograph

1

1.1 General Considerations

The most commonly utilised imaging modality in the evaluation of the skeletal system is conventional radiography (plain film). Technological improvements have led to the use of various modalities, each of which has its own distinct area of superiority. Skeletal radiology is commonly used to diagnose and to treat a wide range of disorders by a variety of health professionals, including medicine, chiropractic, osteopathy, physiotherapy, and podiatry.

X-ray projection depends on the thickness of the tissue that is to be penetrated. When there is no tissue to penetrate, the colour of the picture will be black.

The greater the depth, the lighter the grey.

- Air is projected as black.
- Soft tissues are grey.
- Fluids are a lighter grey.
- Bone is an even lighter grey.
- Metal is projected as white.

1.2 Conventional Radiography

Conventional radiography is the most commonly utilised modality for evaluating bone and joint diseases, particularly traumatic conditions. At least two views of the bone involved, at 90° angles to each other, with each view including two neighbouring joints, should be obtained by the radiologist. This reduces the chances of overlooking a related fracture, subluxation, or dislocation at a site other than the apparent original injury. In youngsters, a radiograph of the normal, unaffected limb is

© The Author(s), under exclusive license to Springer Nature Singapore Pte Ltd. 2023
N. S. Kushwaha, M. B. Abbas, *A Guide to Musculoskeletal Radiology*,
https://doi.org/10.1007/978-981-99-6155-9_1

frequently required for comparison. Standard radiography usually consists of anteroposterior and lateral views; however, oblique and special views are occasionally required, especially when examining complicated structures such as the elbow, knee, wrist, ankle, and pelvis.

1.3   Systematic Reading of X-Rays

Information that should be on the X-ray is:

- Name and age of the patient
- Date of X-ray
- Side of extremity/body

Two views help to fully describe the fracture in both planes. It is easy to miss a fracture with only one view. X-rays of the two adjacent joints must be taken.

1.4   Rule of 2 in Radiography

- 2 Views should be taken, i.e. anteroposterior and lateral view.
- 2 Joints should be spanned, i.e. proximal and distal to the joint involved.
- 2 Sides, i.e. both side radiographs should be taken in immature skeleton because physis can mimic fracture.
- 2 Occasions, i.e. scaphoid fractures.

Using A, B, C, D, E is a helpful and systematic method for musculoskeletal X-ray review:

- A: anatomy and alignment
- B: bone
- C: cartilage
- D: deformity and density
- E: everything else

1.5   Anatomy and Alignment

It is essential to understand the normal anatomy that should be expected for each radiography projection. Knowing what is normal allows you to spot what's not, which is most likely a finding. It's also necessary to be familiar with specific anatomical variations, such as accessory bones.

Alignment should be evaluated to look for dislocations or subluxations, as it will help you spot a dislocated bone in the next steps.

1.5.1   Bone

Bone assessment is the main step of most musculoskeletal radiographs. Check for any signs of fractures; this can usually be done by following along the bone's cortex and recognising any interruptions:

- Follow along the cortex and identify or exclude any interruptions; the cortices should be continuous.
- Check for any lines along the bone; subtle fractures may not interrupt the cortical margin.

1.5.2   Cartilage

Although radiographs do not show cartilage, it serves as a reminder to examine the joints. If the patient is not skeletally mature, the growth cartilages are also examined in this step:

- Examine the articular spaces and note any unusual findings, such as loss of joint space or erosions.
- If the patient's skeleton is immature, don't confuse a physis with a fracture.
- If the patient is skeletally immature, check to see if the predicted ossifications have formed adequately for his or her age. Ossification centres that are underdeveloped or overdeveloped should be noted.

1.5.3   Deformity and Density

If there are no defects, determine if the bone's proper shape has been preserved. Deformities can manifest themselves in a variety of ways, including displaced fractures, bone tumours, bowing, and so on.

Also, consider the density of the bone; X-ray penetration varies between radiographs. One technique to compensate for this is to compare the bone to itself or other bones viewed. Density changes can appear in a variety of ways: localised, widespread, lytic, or sclerotic.

1.5.4   Everything Else

Review everything else, especially soft tissues that were not reviewed in the previous steps. The following are some of the possible findings on a musculoskeletal radiograph:

- Soft tissue swelling
- Lipohaemarthrosis
- Subcutaneous emphysema

1.6   Radiographic Evaluation of Fractures

The following aspects should be included in a full radiographic examination of fractures:

- The anatomic site and extent of a fracture
- The type of fracture, whether incomplete or complete and fracture geometry
- The alignment of the fragments in terms of displacement, angulation, rotation, foreshortening, or distraction
- The direction of the fracture line in relation to the longitudinal axis of the bone
- The presence of special features such as impaction, depression, or compression
- The existence of accompanying abnormalities, such as a fracture with simultaneous dislocation or diastasis
- Unique sorts of fractures that can arise as a result of aberrant stress or as a result of pathologic processes in the bone

   When a fracture is suspected, look for any of the following abnormalities:

- Soft tissue swelling
- Obliteration or displacement of fat stripes
- Joint effusion
- Intracapsular fat–fluid level
- Double cortical line
- Buckling of the cortex
- Irregular metaphyseal corners

   When reporting a fracture, describe (Figs. 1.1, 1.2 and 1.3):

- The side, site, and extent
- The type
- The direction of the fracture line
- The alignment of the fragments
- The presence of impaction, depression, or compression
- The presence of associated abnormalities
- Whether the fracture is a special type
- Whether the growth plate is involved (Salter-Harris classification)

Fig. 1.1 Fracture shaft of femur

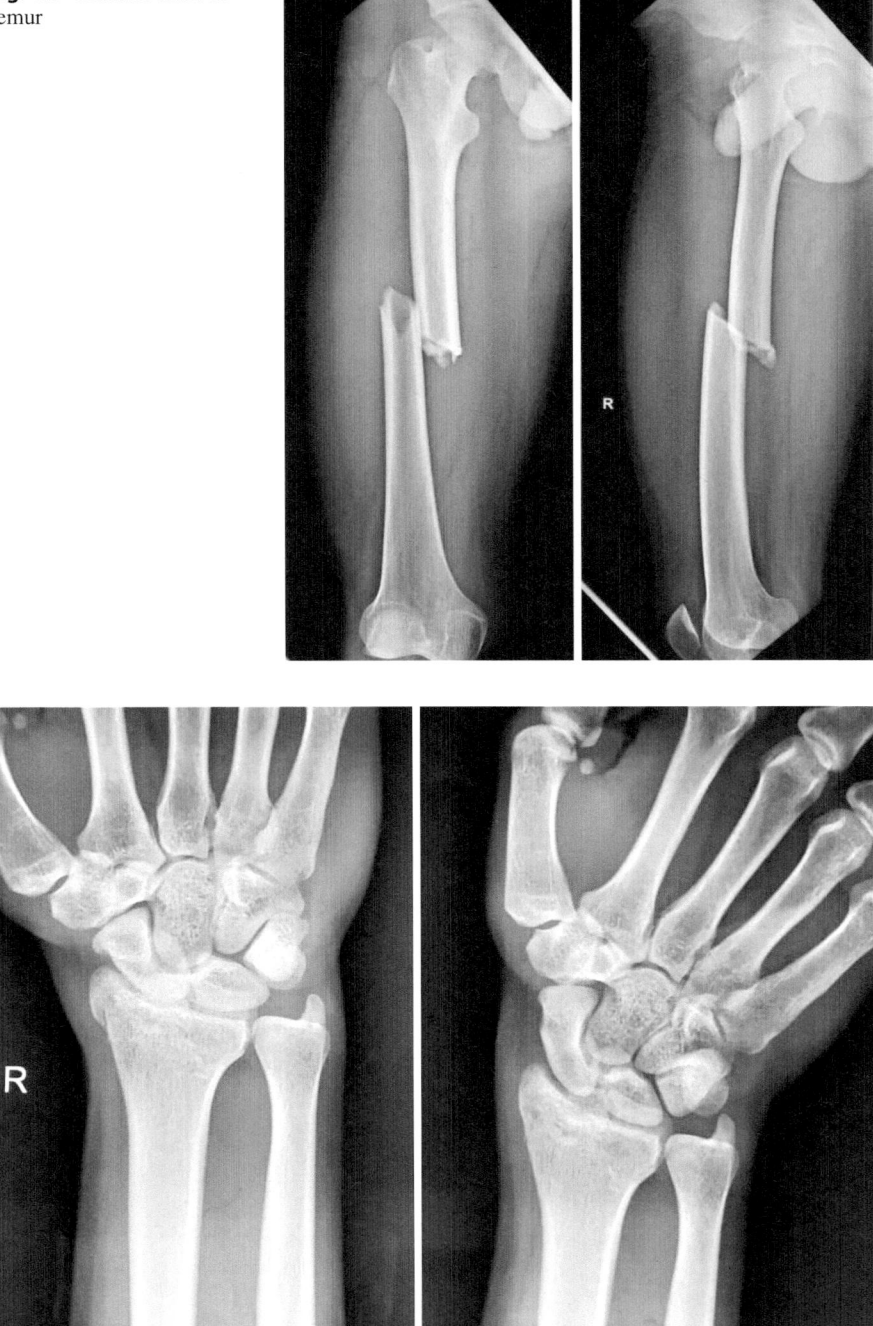

Fig. 1.2 AP and scaphoid view of wrist joint

Fig. 1.3 X-Ray pelvis
with bilateral hip AP view

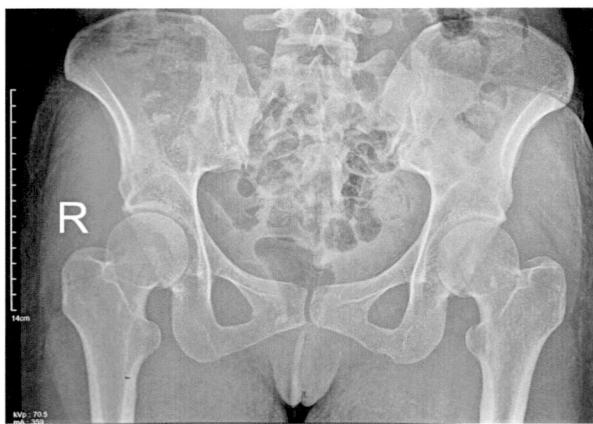

1.7   Fracture Healing and Complications

The patient's age, the site and kind of fracture, the position of the fragments, the
state of the blood supply, the quality of immobilisation or fixation, and the presence
or absence of accompanying abnormalities such as infection or osteonecrosis are all
factors that influence fracture healing. The majority of fractures heal through a combination of endosteal and periosteal callus formation. Undisplaced fractures and
anatomically reduced fractures immobilised with enough compression heal via primary union if the blood supply is adequate. The fracture line is obliterated by endosteal (internal) callus in this kind of healing. Secondary union heals displaced
fractures, or those that are not anatomically aligned or have a gap between fragments. Excessive periosteal (external) callus, which undergoes full ossification
through the stages of granulation tissue, fibrous tissue, fibrocartilage, woven bone,
and compact bone, is responsible for this form of healing. The radiologist should be
aware of radiographic signs of related healing difficulties in addition to monitoring
the course of callus formation. Delayed union, nonunion, and malunion are examples of problems (Fig. 1.4).

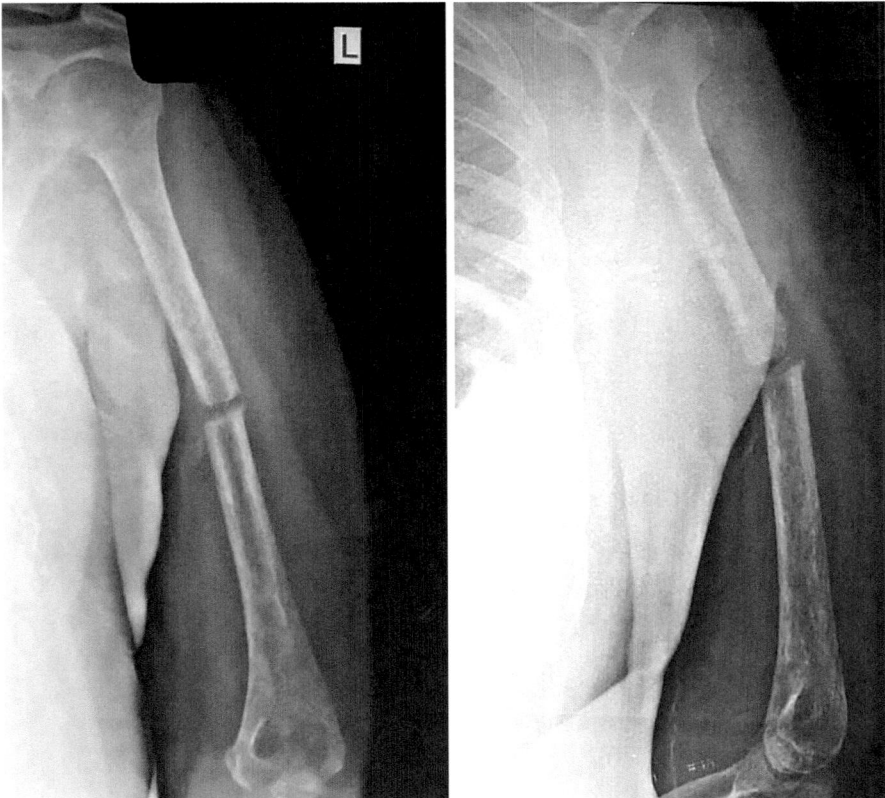

Fig. 1.4 Nonunion of shaft of humerus

1.8   Radiographic Evaluation of Arthritides

Arthritis, in its broadest sense, refers to a joint abnormality caused by a degenerative, inflammatory, viral, or metabolic process. Connective tissue arthropathies, such as those linked with systemic lupus erythematosus (SLE) and scleroderma, are also classified among the arthritides. Conventional radiography is the most significant technique for evaluating arthritis. Standard radiographs of the affected joint should be acquired in at least two projections at 90° to each other, as in the radiographic examination of traumatic situations. A weight-bearing view may be useful, especially for a dynamic assessment of any reduction in joint space caused by the body's weight. Special projections may be required at times to indicate damaging changes in the joint in order to gain a competitive advantage (Figs. 1.5 and 1.6).

Fig. 1.5 Bilateral
inflammatory arthritis of
hip joint

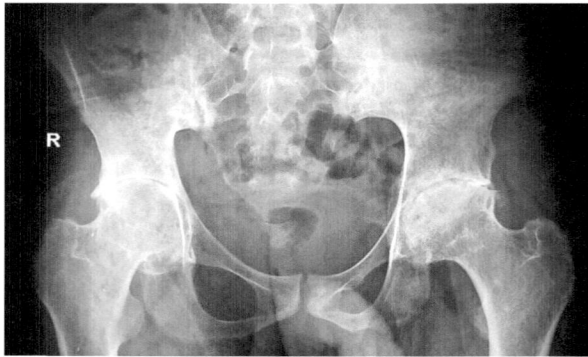

Fig. 1.6 Degenerative
osteoarthritis of knee joint

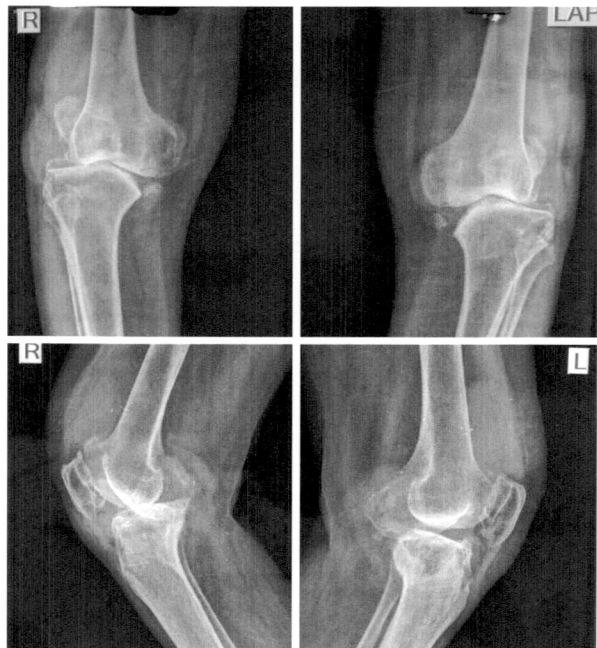

1.9   Radiographic Evaluation of Tumour and Tumour-Like Lesions

The typical radiographic images relevant to the anatomic site under inquiry are usually sufficient to make a proper diagnosis, which can then be verified by biopsy and histopathologic evaluation. The most helpful information on the location and shape of a lesion comes from conventional radiography, especially when it comes to the kind of bone damage, calcifications, ossifications, and periosteal reaction.

The age of the patient, the duration of the symptoms, and the tumour's growth rate are the most useful clinical data for patients with suspected bone or soft tissue lesions.

Several critical radiographic features should be examined when evaluating tumours or tumour-like bone lesions, including:

- Lesion's location (the particular bone and site in the bone affected)
- Type of the lesion's border (narrow or wide zone of transition)
- Type of bone damage (calcified, ossified, or hollow)
- Type of matrix (calcified, ossified, or hollow) (geographic, moth-eaten, or permeative)
- Presence or absence of soft tissue extension (sunburst, velvet, lamellated, Codman triangle)
- The periosteal reaction (solid or interrupted—sunburst, velvet, lamellated, Codman triangle)

A lesion most likely represents a benign tumour when it exhibits:

- Geographic bone destruction
- A sclerotic margin
- Solid, uninterrupted periosteal reaction, or no periosteal response
- No soft tissue mass
  A lesion most likely represents a malignant tumour when it shows:
- Poorly defined margins (a wide zone of transition)
- A moth-eaten or permeative type of bone destruction
- An interrupted periosteal reaction
- A soft tissue mass

A lesion most likely represents a cartilage tumour (e.g. enchondroma or chondrosarcoma) when it exhibits:

- Lobulation (endosteal scalloping)
- Punctate, annular, or comma-like calcifications in the matrix

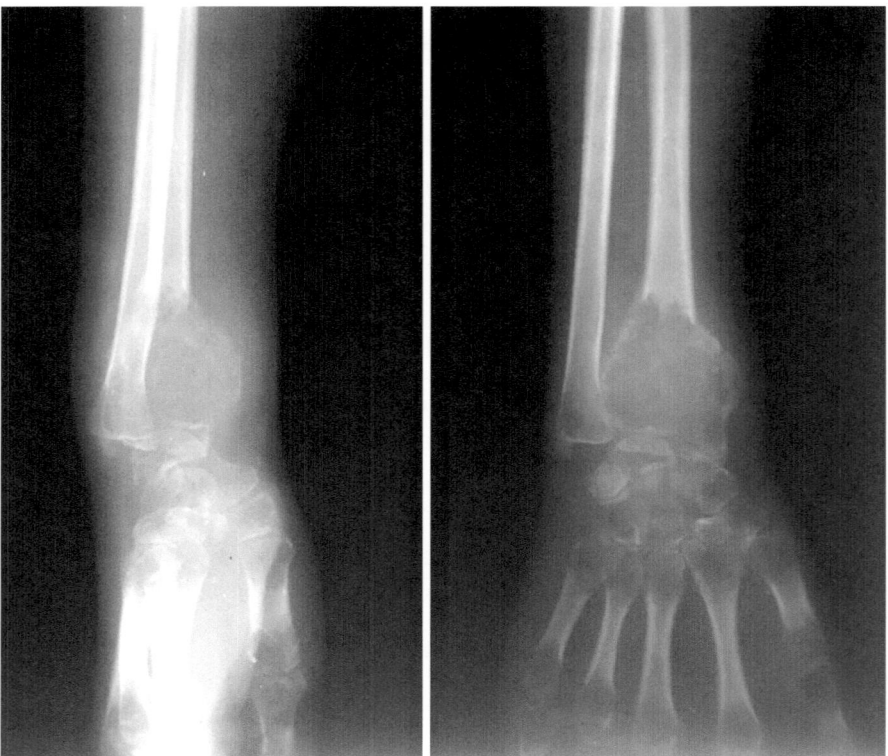

Expansile lytic lesion in epiphysio-metaphyseal region of distal end of radius with thinning and ballooning of cortex and multiple septations in a mature skeleton suggesting benign bony lesion (giant cell tumour).

1.10   Radiographic Evaluation of Musculoskeletal Infections

Most of the time, radiography is enough to show the relevant signs of a bone or joint infection. Magnification radiography was once useful for identifying tiny changes that could indicate cortical loss or periosteal new bone growth (Figs. 1.7 and 1.8).

The imaging hallmarks of osteomyelitis include:

- Cortical and medullary bone destruction
- Reactive sclerosis and a periosteal reaction
- The presence of sequestra and involucra

The radiographic hallmarks of tuberculous infection of an intervertebral disk are:

- Narrowing of the disk space
- Loss of the sharp outline of the adjacent vertebral end plates

Fig. 1.7 Chronic osteomyelitis of shaft of femur showing sequestrum formation

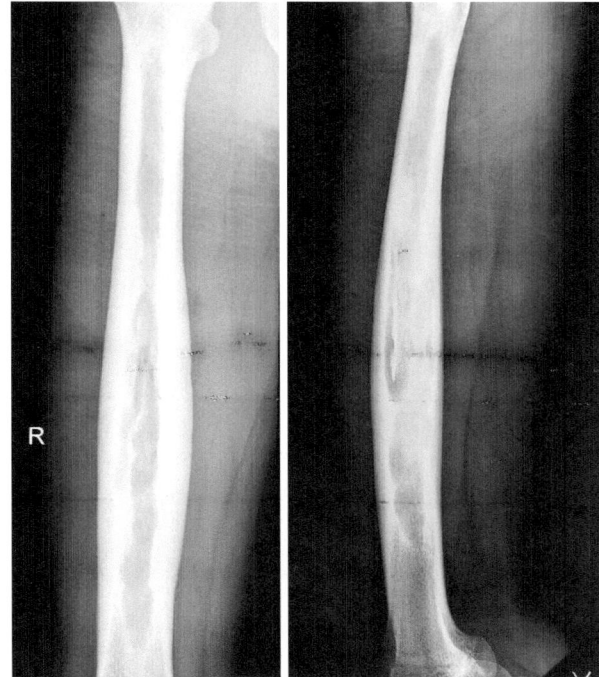

Tuberculous infection of the spine may:

- Destroy the disk and vertebra, leading to kyphosis and a gibbus formation
- Extend into the soft tissues, forming a cold abscess

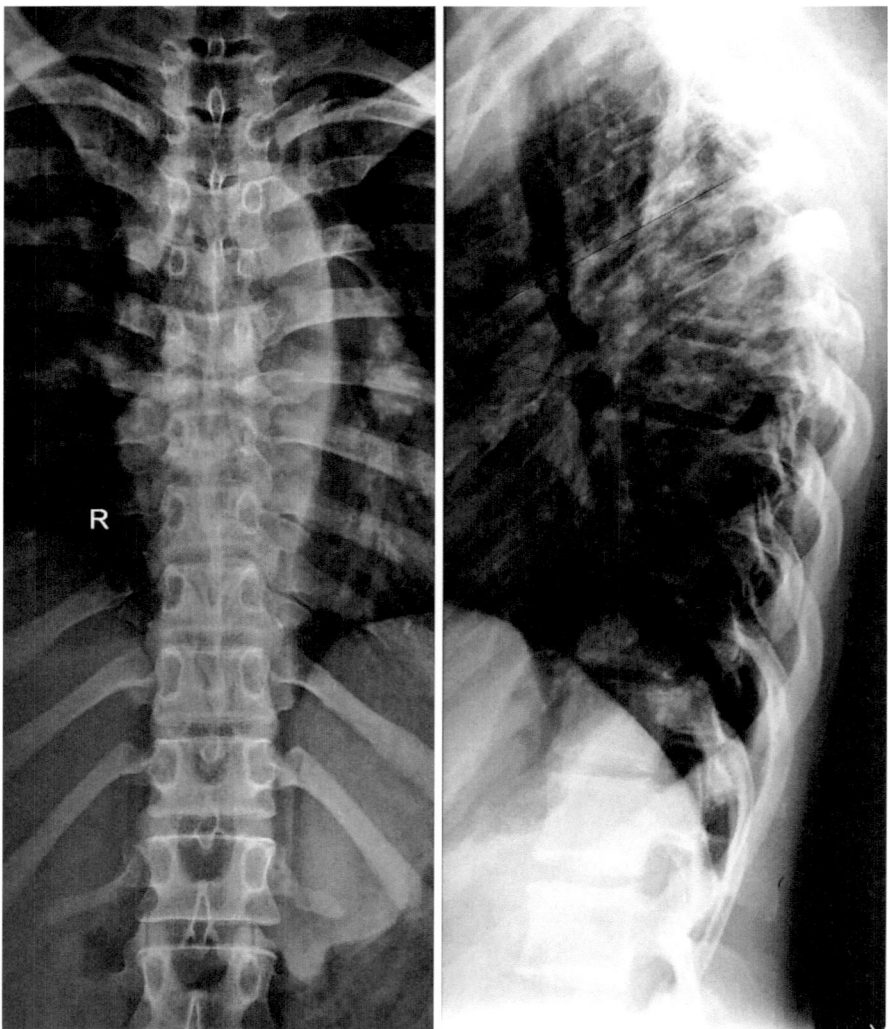

Fig. 1.8 AP and lateral view of dorso-lumbar spine showing destruction and collapse of D6–D7 vertebrae, decreased IV disc space with bird's nest abscess (Pott's spine)

1.11   Radiographic Evaluation of Metabolic and Endocrine Disorders

The simplest and most extensively used method of determining bone density is radiography. This approach can identify even tiny increases in bone density, but it usually fails to detect losses in overall skeletal mineralisation unless the reduction is more than 30%. It should be noted that technical faults, such as incorrect kilovoltage and milliamperage settings, can readily cause normal bone to have an aberrant radiographic image. Overexposure, for example, appears to enhance bone radiolucency, whereas underexposure appears to increase bone radiodensity artificially. Increased bone radiolucency (osteopenia) or increased bone density (osteosclerosis) on a routine radiograph is linked to the process of bone formation and resorption, which is normally in balance:

- If bone resorption exceeds bone production, either due to an increase in osteoclast activity or a decrease in osteoblast activity, or due to insufficient mineral deposition in the matrix, the result is increased radiolucency of the bone.
- If bone production exceeds bone resorption, either due to an increase in osteoblast activity or a decrease in osteoclast activity, the result is increased radiodensity of the bone.

1.12   Shoulder

See Figs. 1.9, 1.10, and 1.11.

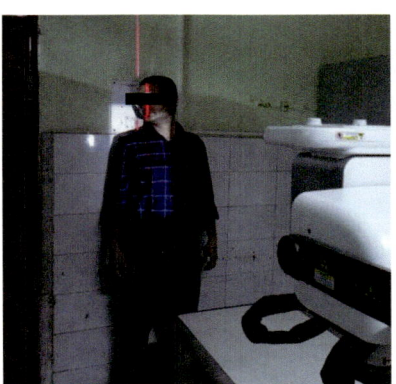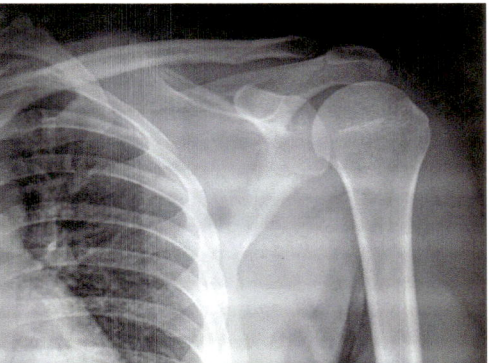

Fig. 1.9 AP view of shoulder joint

Fig. 1.10 Axillary view of shoulder joint

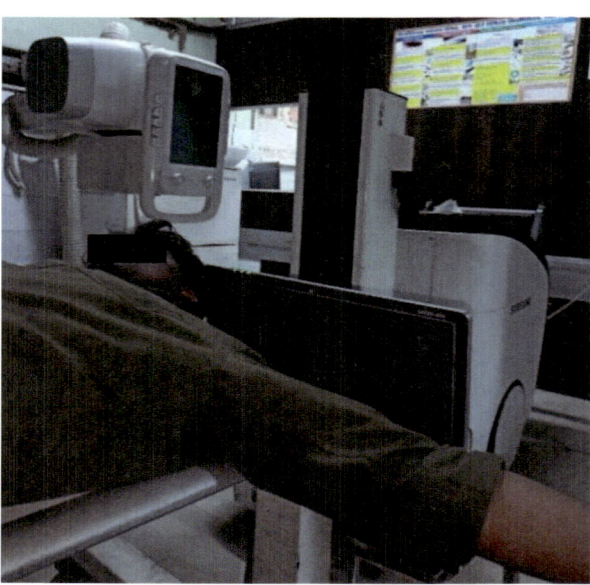

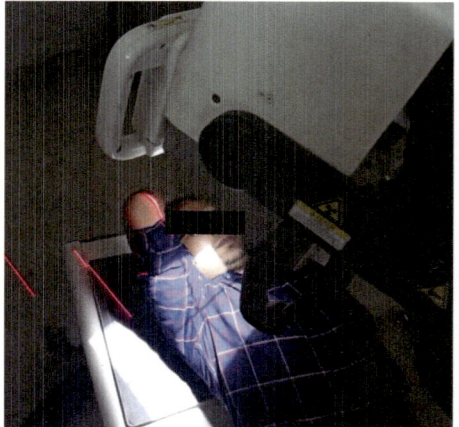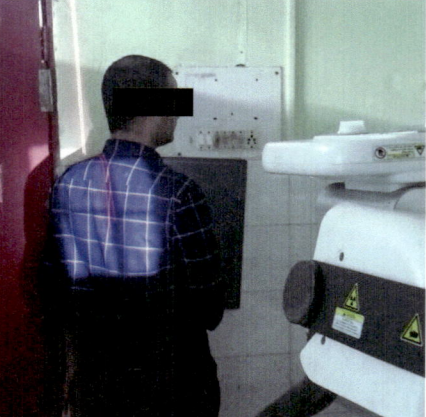

Fig. 1.11 Stryker notch view and Scapular Y view

1.13   Cervical Spine (Fig. 1.12)

- Count the vertebrae
- Adequacy (all cervical vertebrae visualised or not)
- Modified views (views with increased penetration, with traction of arm, swimmers view, oblique views)
- Detect the rotation of spine

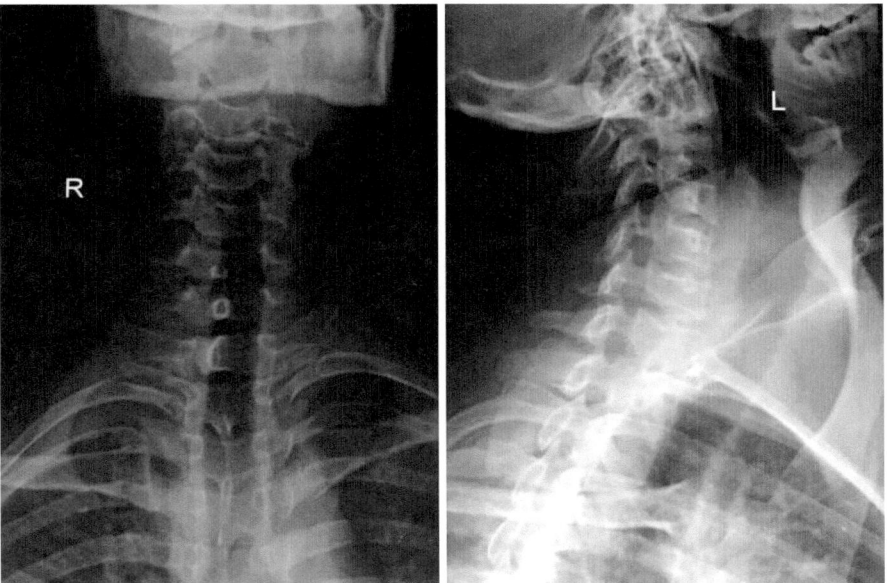

Fig. 1.12 Normal X-ray of cervical spine

1.14   The Acetabulum

Iliac oblique: 45° anterior rotation of unaffected side

- Anterior wall
- Posterior column
- Ilioischial line

Obturator oblique: 45° anterior rotation of affected side (only obturator oblique view show obturator foramen) (Figs. 1.13, 1.14, and 1.15)

- Posterior wall
- Anterior column
- Iliopectineal line

Fig. 1.13 Judet view for acetabulum

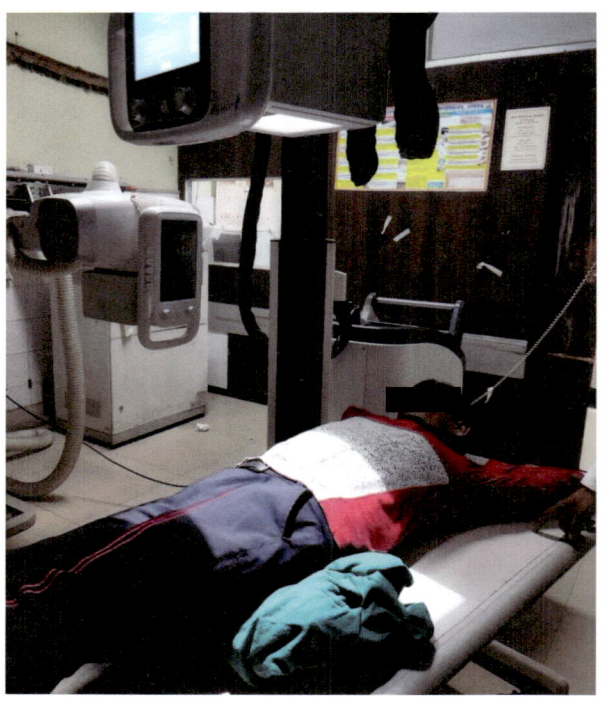

Fig. 1.14 Iliac oblique view of left acetabulum

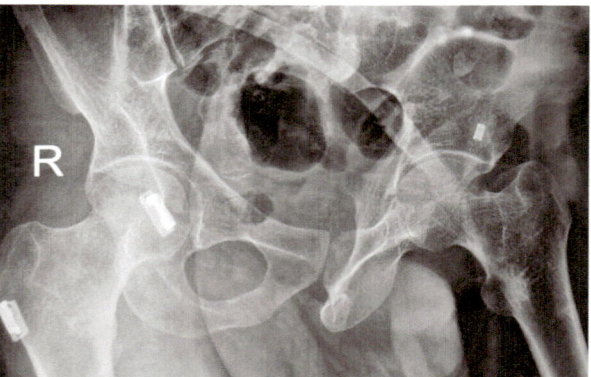

Fig. 1.15 Obturator view of left acetabulum

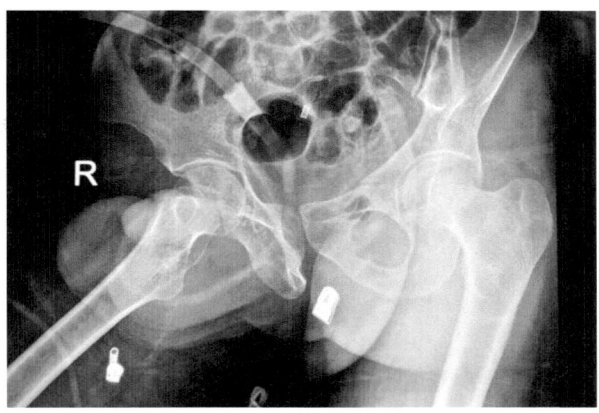

1.15   The Ankle Joint

See Figs. 1.16, 1.17, 1.18, and 1.19.

Fig. 1.16 AP view

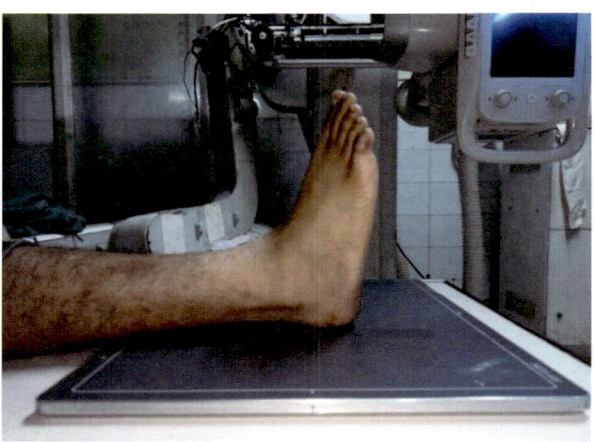

Fig. 1.17 Mortise view
(taken with the foot in
15–20° of internal rotation
to offset the intermalleolar
axis)

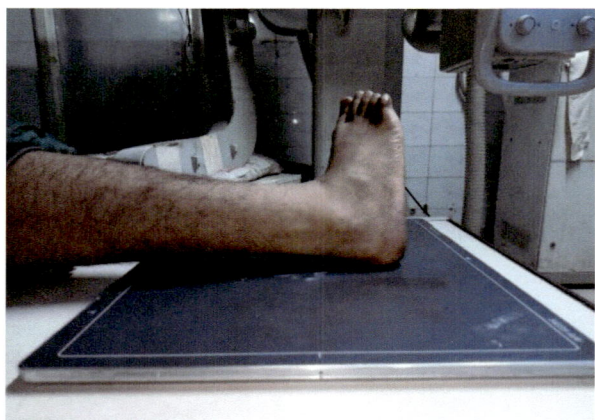

Fig. 1.18 Lateral view
(fibular shadow overlap
posterior part of tibia)

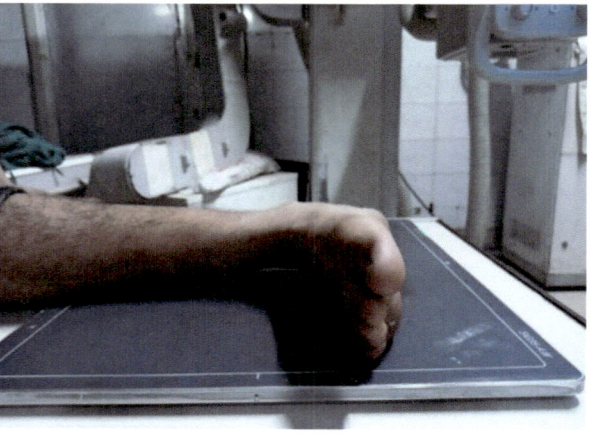

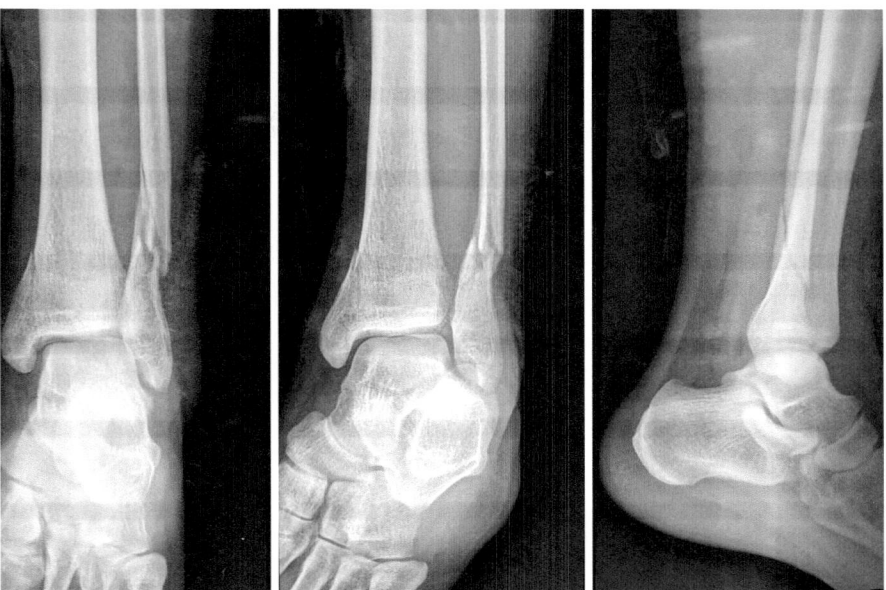

Fig. 1.19 AP, Mortise, and Lateral view of ankle joint showing Bimalleolar fracture

1.16   Patella

See Fig. 1.20.

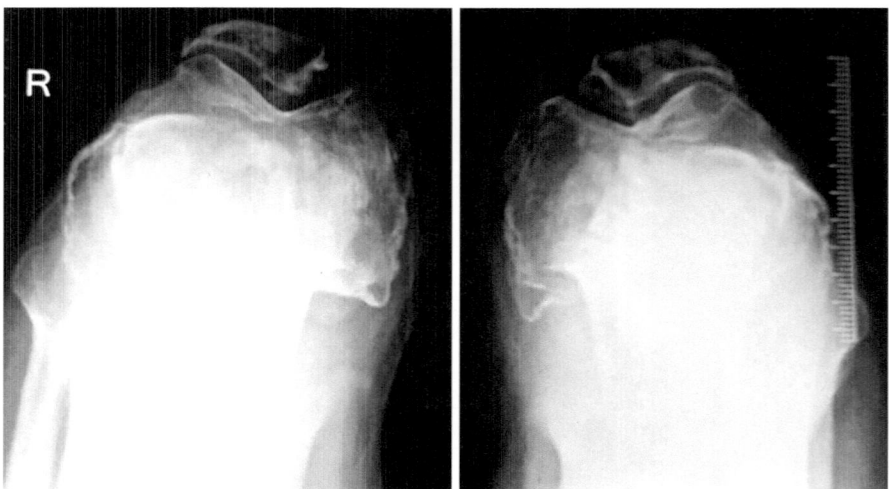

Fig. 1.20 Skyline view of patella

Bibliography

1. Nelson SW. Some important diagnostic and technical fundamentals in the radiology of trauma, with particular emphasis on skeletal trauma. *Radiol Clin North Am* 1966;4:241–259.
2. Naimark A, Miller K, Segal D, Kossoff J. Nonunion. *Skeletal Radiol* 1981;6:21–25.
3. Rogers LF. *Radiology of skeletal trauma*. New York: Churchill Livingstone; 1992.

Part II

Musculoskeletal Trauma

Radiographs of Upper Extremity: Fractures and Dislocations

2

Dislocation of a joint is an orthopaedic emergency. Every clinician must read the radiograph for its prompt diagnosis. Shoulder joint is the commonest of all dislocations.

2.1 Shoulder Dislocation

The shoulder, which accounts for up to 45% of all dislocations, is the most often dislocated major joint in the body. Ninety-six percent of cases involve anterior dislocations. The second most common type of dislocation is posterior dislocation, which accounts for 2–4% of occurrences. Shoulder dislocations, both inferior (luxatio erecta) and superior (luxatio erecta), are uncommon, accounting for just around 0.5% of occurrences (Fig. 2.1).

Classification:

Degree of stability: Dislocation versus subluxation
Chronology: Congenital acute versus chronic
Locked (fixed)
Recurrent
Acquired: generally from repeated minor injuries (swimming, gymnastics, weights); labrum often intact but with capsular laxity; increased glenohumeral joint volume; subluxation common
Force: Atraumatic: usually owing to congenital laxity; no injury; often asymptomatic; self-reducing
Traumatic: usually caused by one major injury; anterior or inferior labrum may be detached (Bankart lesion); unidirectional; generally requires assistance for reduction

© The Author(s), under exclusive license to Springer Nature Singapore Pte
Ltd. 2023
N. S. Kushwaha, M. B. Abbas, *A Guide to Musculoskeletal Radiology*,
https://doi.org/10.1007/978-981-99-6155-9_2

Fig. 2.1 Anterior shoulder dislocation. AP radiograph of shoulder showing humeral head is outside the glenoid cavity and lies beneath the inferior rim of glenoid

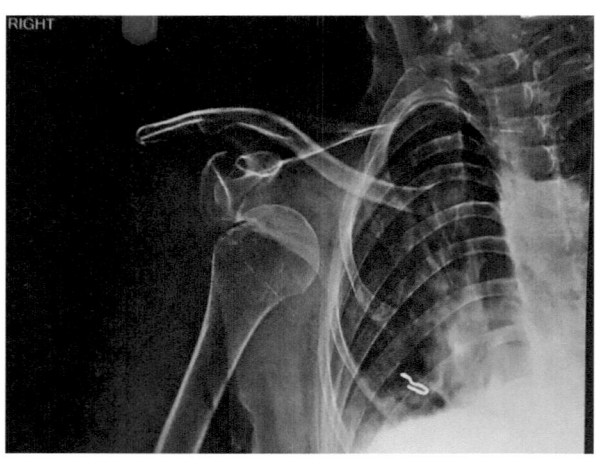

Patient contribution: Voluntary versus involuntary
Direction: Subcoracoid
Subglenoid
Intrathoracic

2.2   Scapula Fracture

A trauma series of the shoulder, consisting of a true anteroposterior view, an axillary view, and a Scapular-Y view (true scapular lateral), should be taken first; these should be able to show most glenoid, scapular neck, body, and acromion fractures (Fig. 2.2).

Fig. 2.2 AP radiograph of shoulder showing fracture neck of scapula

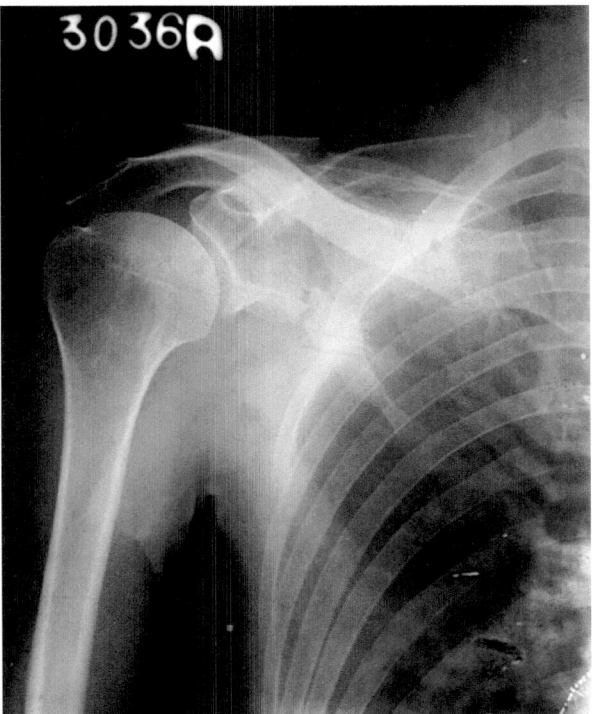

2.3   Acromioclavicular Joint Disruption

See Fig. 2.3.

Fig. 2.3 AP radiograph of
shoulder showing
acromioclavicular joint
disruption of right shoulder

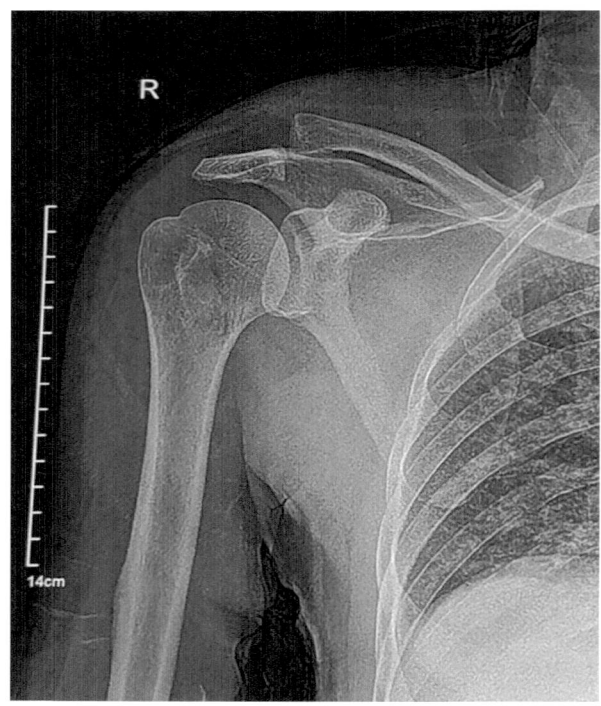

2.4   Proximal Humerus Fractures

Proximal humerus fractures account for 4–5% of all humerus fractures and are the most prevalent type of humerus fracture (45%) (Figs. 2.4 and 2.5).

Fracture types include:

- **One-part fractures**: No displaced fragments regardless of number of fracture lines
- **Two-part fractures** (any of the following):
  - Anatomic neck
  - Surgical neck
  - Greater tuberosity
  - Lesser tuberosity
- **Three-part fractures**:
  - Surgical neck with greater tuberosity
  - Surgical neck with lesser tuberosity
- **Four-part fractures**
- **Fracture dislocation**
- **Articular surface fracture**

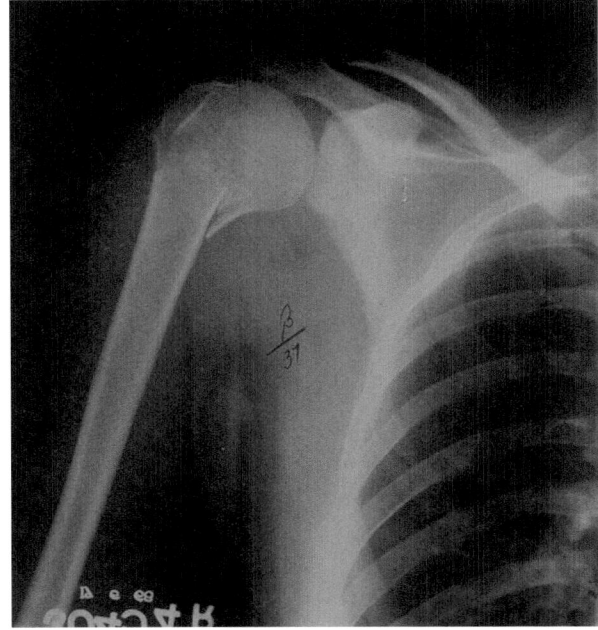

Fig. 2.4 Fracture of proximal humerus. Anteroposterior radiograph of the shoulder demonstrates a comminuted fracture through the surgical neck of the humerus

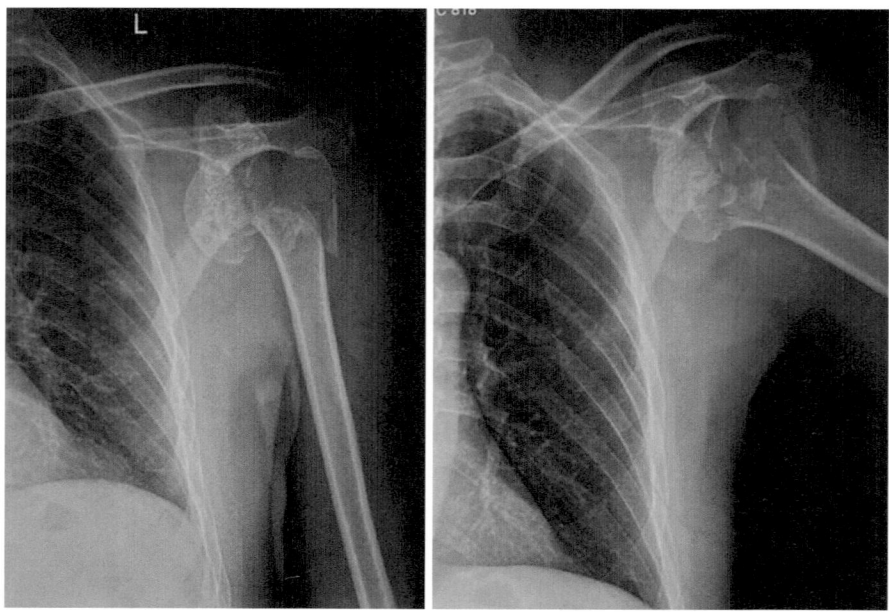

Fig. 2.5 Anteroposterior radiograph of the shoulder demonstrates a four-part fracture of surgical neck humerus

2.5   Fracture Shaft Humerus

See Fig. 2.6.

Fig. 2.6 AP and lateral radiograph of arm showing transverse fracture shaft humerus (mid one-third)

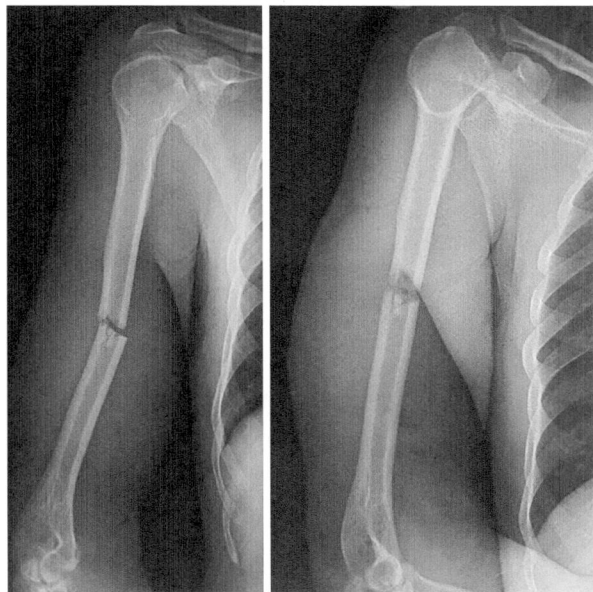

2.6   Intercondylar Humerus Fracture

Obtain standard anteroposterior (AP) and lateral images of the elbow. For further fracture definition, oblique radiographs may be useful. Traction radiographs can help with preoperative planning by better delineating the fracture pattern (Fig. 2.7).

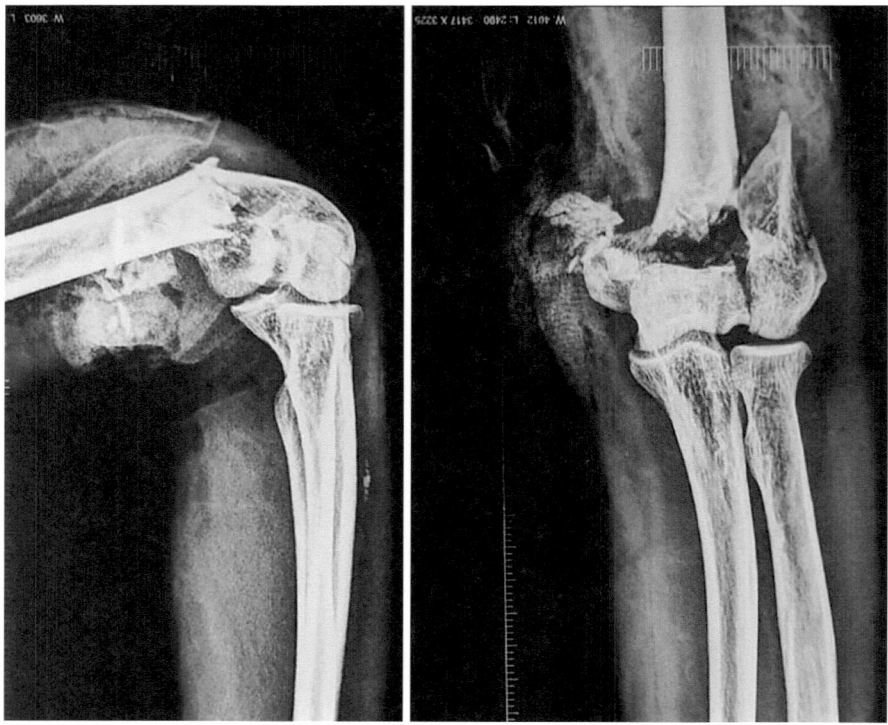

Fig. 2.7   AP and lateral radiograph of elbow showing intercondylar fracture distal humerus

2.7   Olecranon Fracture

See Fig. 2.8.

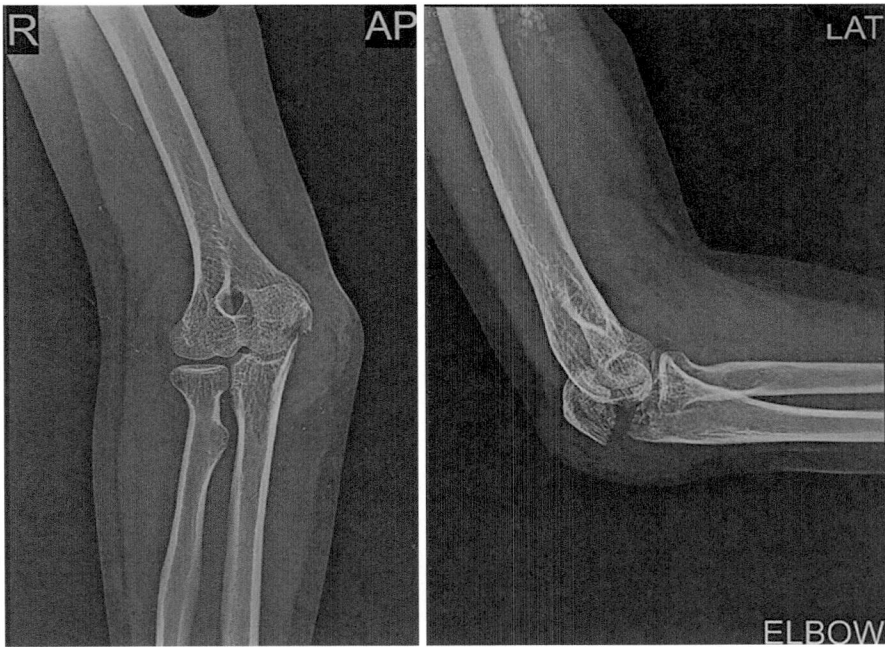

Fig. 2.8 AP and lateral radiograph of elbow showing transverse fracture of olecranon

2.8   Elbow Dislocation

Elbow dislocation occurs in 11–28% of all elbow injuries. The most common type of elbow dislocation is posterior dislocation, which accounts for 80–90% of all elbow dislocations.

Obtain standard anteroposterior and lateral radiographs of the elbow. The ulno-humeral and radiocapitellar joints should be checked for congruency. Radiographs of the elbow should be examined for concomitant fractures. Valgus stress images acquired after first reduction or after surgery at 30 degrees' elbow flexion and full forearm pronation may aid in the diagnosis of an MCL injury (Fig. 2.9).

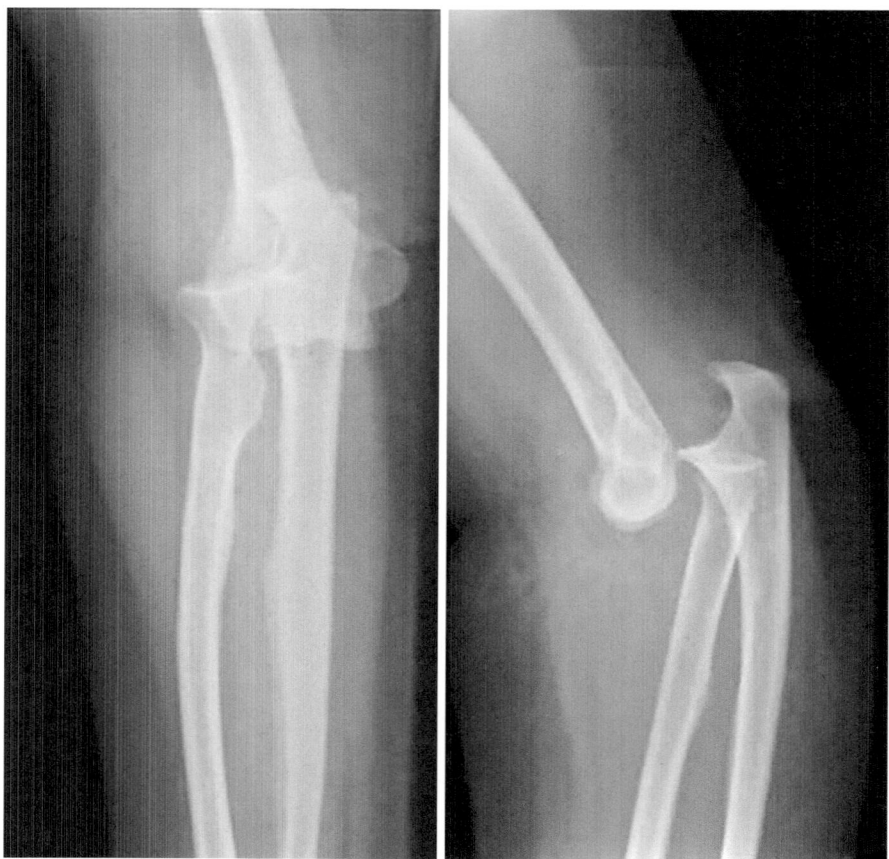

Fig. 2.9   AP and lateral radiograph of elbow showing posterior dislocation

2.9   **Radial Head Fracture**

Oblique views (Greenspan view) should be obtained in cases where a fracture is suspected but not visible on AP and lateral views. With the forearm in neutral rotation and the radiography beam tilted 45° cephalad, a Greenspan view is obtained, which allows imaging of the radiocapitellar articulation (Fig. 2.10).

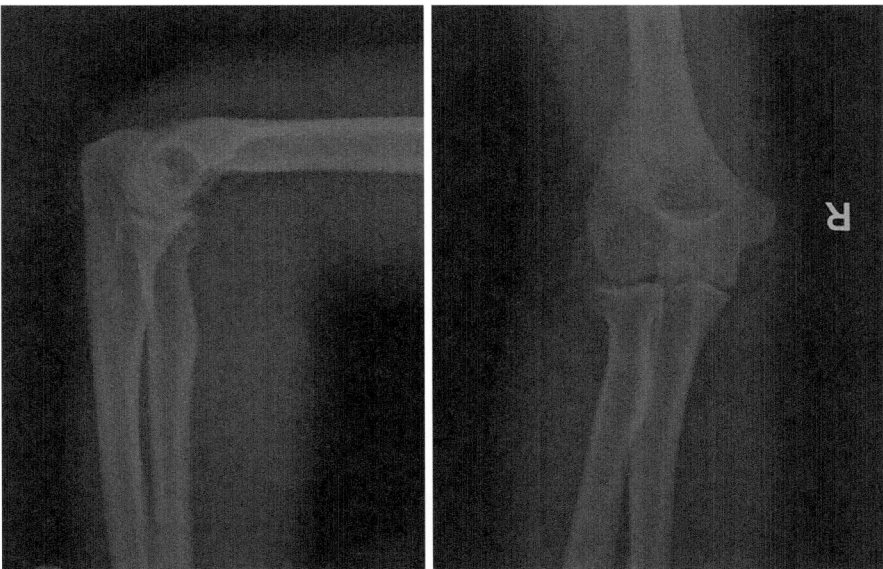

Fig. 2.10   AP and lateral radiograph of elbow showing fracture radial head

2.10   Monteggia Fracture Dislocation

A Monteggia lesion is defined as a proximal ulna fracture with radial head dislocation.

2.11   Bado Classification

Type I: Anterior dislocation of the radial head with fracture of ulnar diaphysis at any level with anterior angulation

Type II: Posterior/posterolateral dislocation of the radial head with fracture of ulnar diaphysis with posterior angulation

Type III: Lateral/anterolateral dislocation of the radial head with fracture of ulnar metaphysis

Type IV: Anterior dislocation of the radial head with fractures of both radius and ulna within proximal third at the same level

The forearm must be seen from the AP and lateral perspectives (additional views should cover the wrist and elbow). Fracture definition could be aided by oblique views. Findings on a normal X-ray: The capitellum should always line up with a line drawn through the radial head and shaft. Supinated lateral: The capitellum should be encircled by lines drawn tangential to the radial head anteriorly and posteriorly (Fig. 2.11).

Fig. 2.11 AP and lateral radiograph of forearm showing fracture proximal ulna with radial head dislocation (Monteggia fracture dislocation)

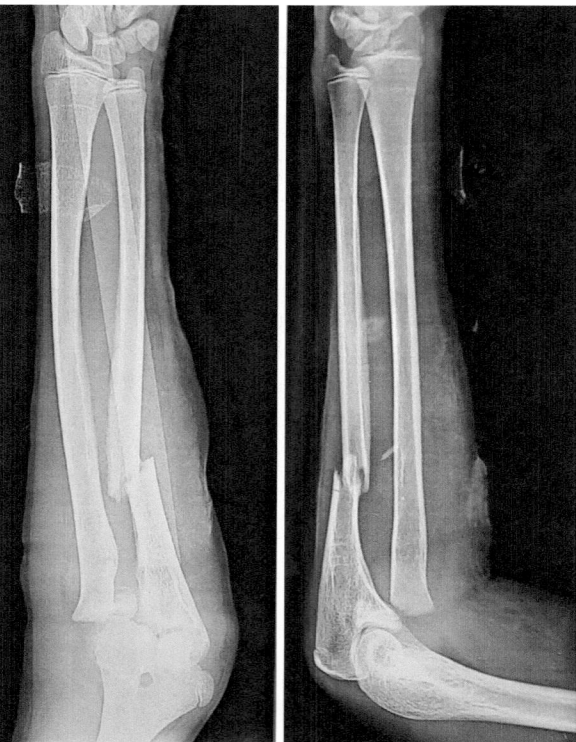

2.12   Galeazzi Fracture Dislocation

A Galeazzi fracture is a distal radioulnar joint disruption caused by a fracture of the radial diaphysis at the junction of the middle and distal thirds. Because it necessitates open reduction and internal fixation, it is also known as the "fracture of necessity" (Fig. 2.12).

Radiographic signs of distal radioulnar joint injury are:

- Fracture at base of the ulnar styloid
- Widened distal radioulnar joint on AP X-ray
- Subluxed ulna on lateral X-ray
- >5-mm radial shortening

Fig. 2.12 AP and lateral radiograph of forearm with wrist showing fracture distal one-third radius with distal radioulnar joint disruption (Galeazzi fracture dislocation)

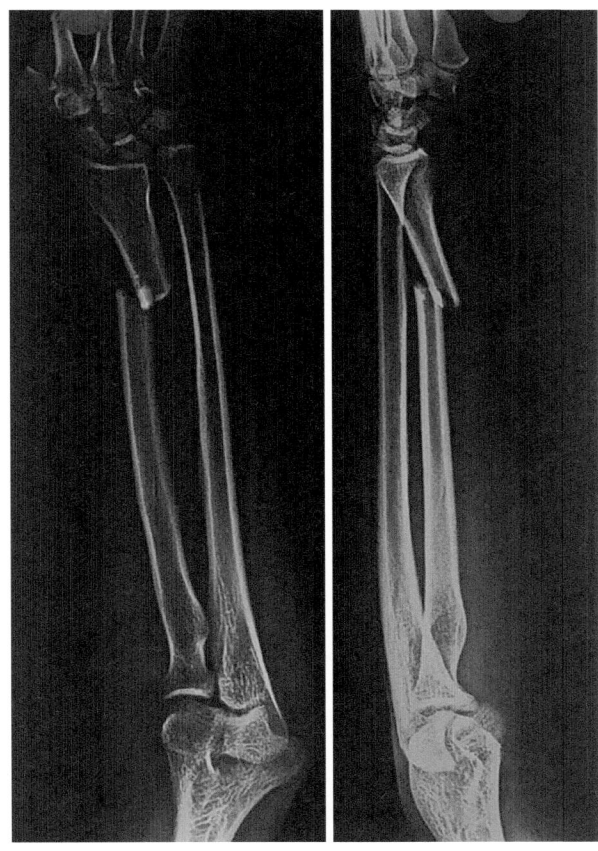

2.13   Distal Radius Fractures

Distal radius fractures are among the most common upper extremity fractures. Distal radius fractures account for nearly a sixth of all fractures treated in emergency rooms and around 16% of all fractures treated by orthopaedic surgeons.

If necessary, take AP and lateral views of the wrist, as well as oblique views for additional fracture definition. The patient's normal ulnar variance and scapholunate angle can be assessed using contralateral wrist views (Fig. 2.13).

Normal radiographic relationships:

- **Radial inclination:** averages 23° (range, 13–30°)
- **Radial length:** averages 11 mm (range, 8–18 mm)
- **Palmar (volar) tilt:** averages 11–12° (range, 0–28°)

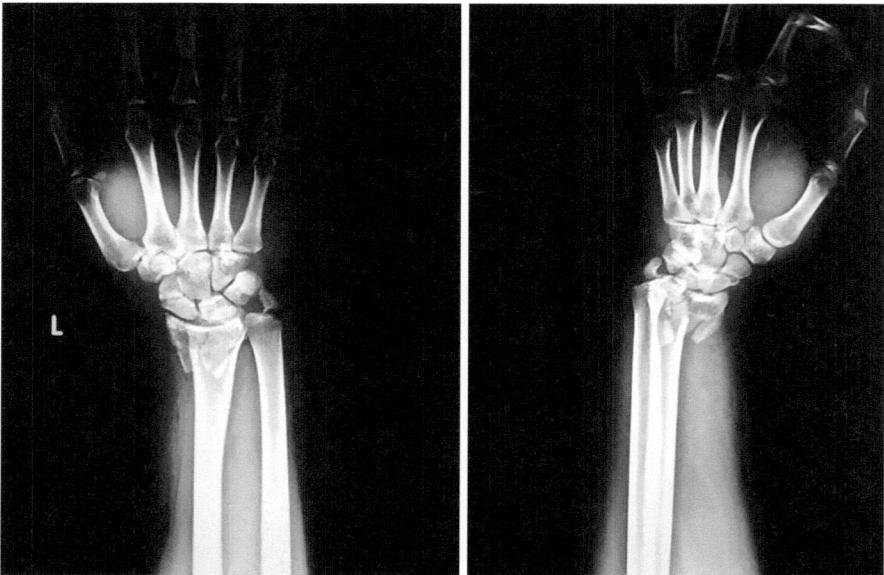

Fig. 2.13 AP and lateral radiograph of wrist showing comminuted intra-articular fracture of distal end radius (Volar Barton type)

2.14   Scaphoid Fracture

Fractures of the scaphoid are common and account for about 50–80% of carpal injuries.

AP view of the wrist in ulnar deviation, a lateral, a supinated AP and pronated oblique view, and a clenched supinated view in ulnar deviation are all used in radiographic evaluation. In up to 25% of instances, initial films are nondiagnostic. If the clinical examination suggests fracture but radiographs are negative, an immobilisation trial with follow-up radiographs 1–2 weeks after injury may reveal the fracture (Fig. 2.14).

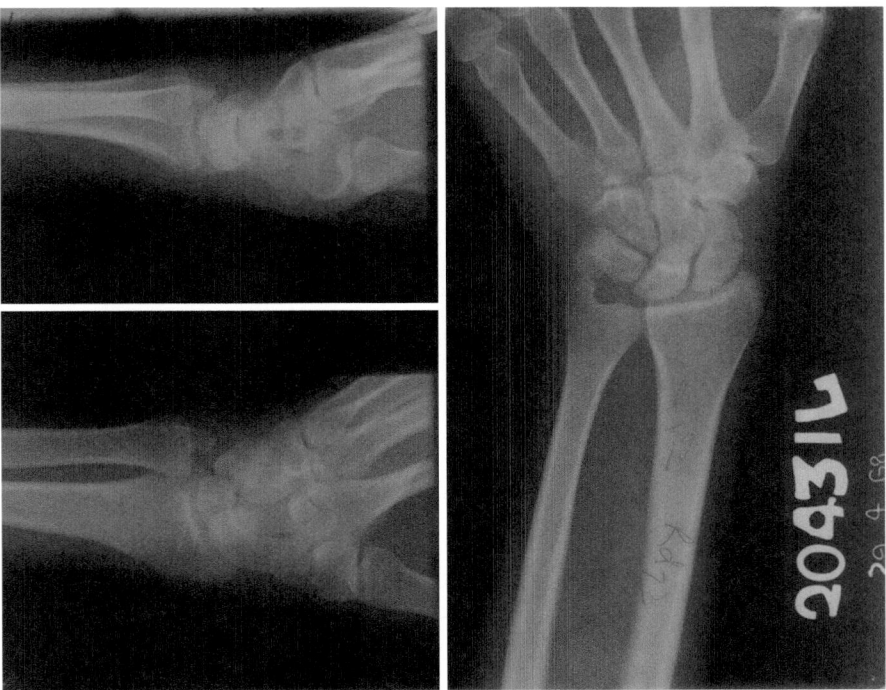

Fig. 2.14 AP, lateral, and scaphoid radiograph of wrist showing fracture waist of scaphoid

2.15   Metacarpal Fracture

A radiograph of the affected digit or hand should be taken from the back, side, and oblique positions. To avoid overlapping of other digits over the area of interest, injured digits should be examined individually (Fig. 2.15).

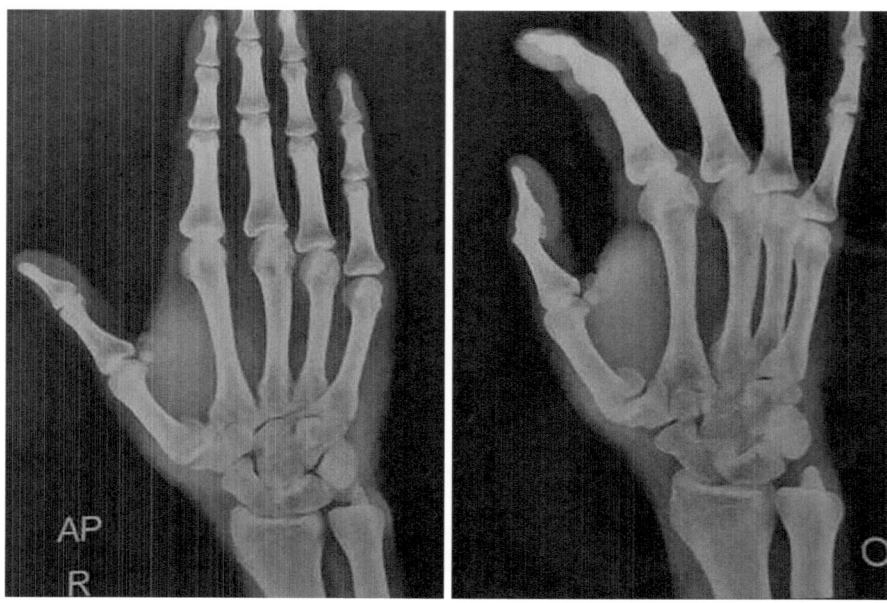

Fig. 2.15 AP and oblique radiograph of hand shows intra-articular fracture base of first metacarpal (Bennet fracture)

Bibliography

1. Greenspan A Beltran J. *Orthopedic Imaging: A Practical Approach.* Sixth ed. Philadelphia: Wolters Kluwer; 2015.
2. Egol KA Koval KJ Zuckerman JD Ovid Technologies Inc. *Handbook of Fractures.* Fifth ed. Philadelphia: Wolters Kluwer Health; 2015.

Radiographs of Lower Extremity: Fractures and Dislocations

3

3.1 Hip Dislocation

Hip dislocations are the second most common joint dislocation after shoulder. Dislocation can be posterior (commonest), central, or anterior. The femoral heads should appear similar in size and the joint spaces should be symmetric across the pelvis on AP view. The affected femoral head appears smaller than the normal femoral head in posterior dislocations. The femoral head appears to be significantly larger in anterior dislocation. The Shenton line should be intact and smooth. The appearance of the greater and lesser trochanters in relation to one another could indicate pathologic internal or external hip rotation. The femoral shaft should also be observed in its adducted or abducted position. Before attempting any manipulative reduction, a thorough examination of the femoral neck is required to rule out the presence of a femoral neck fracture (Figs. 3.1 and 3.2).

© The Author(s), under exclusive license to Springer Nature Singapore Pte Ltd. 2023
N. S. Kushwaha, M. B. Abbas, *A Guide to Musculoskeletal Radiology*,
https://doi.org/10.1007/978-981-99-6155-9_3

Fig. 3.1 Posterior hip dislocation. X-ray pelvis with both hip AP view shows break in Shenton's line, head of femur out of acetabulum and overlapping the supra-acetabular area with fracture of posterior wall of acetabulum. Femur is adducted and internally rotated

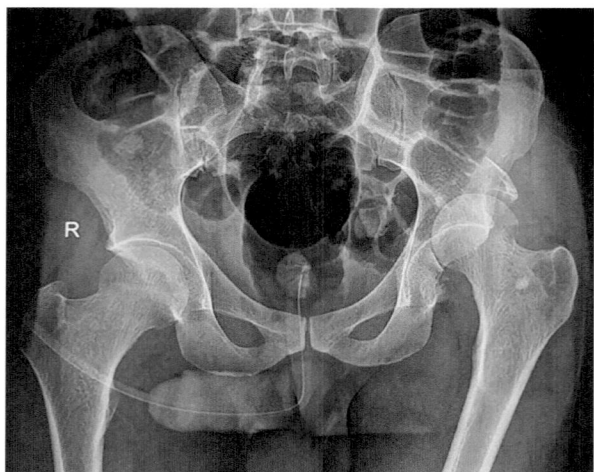

Fig. 3.2 Anterior hip dislocation. X-ray pelvis with both hip AP view shows break in Shenton's line, head of femur out of acetabulum and overlapping the ischium

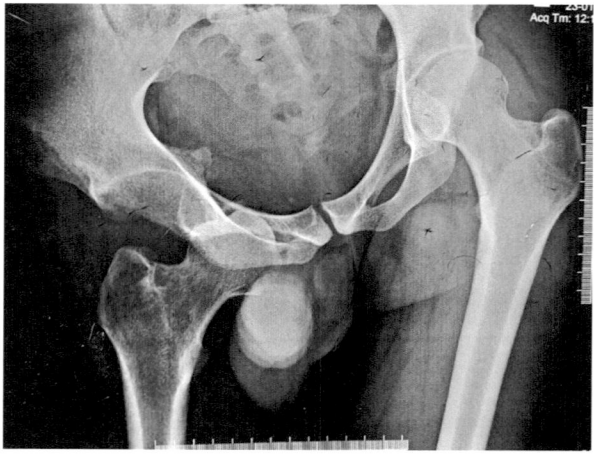

3.2   Fracture Neck Femur

Incidence is bimodal. Younger individuals have a relatively low incidence of this fracture, which is mostly linked to high-energy trauma. Low-energy falls cause the vast majority of fractures in the elderly (Fig. 3.3).

Garden classification is based on the degree of displacement.

Type I: Incomplete/valgus impacted.
Type II: Complete and undisplaced on AP and lateral views.
Type III: Complete with partial displacement; trabecular pattern of the femoral head does not line up with that of the acetabulum.
Type IV: Completely displaced; trabecular pattern of the head assumes a parallel orientation with that of the acetabulum.

Fig. 3.3   X-ray pelvis with both hip AP view shows completely displaced fracture neck femur

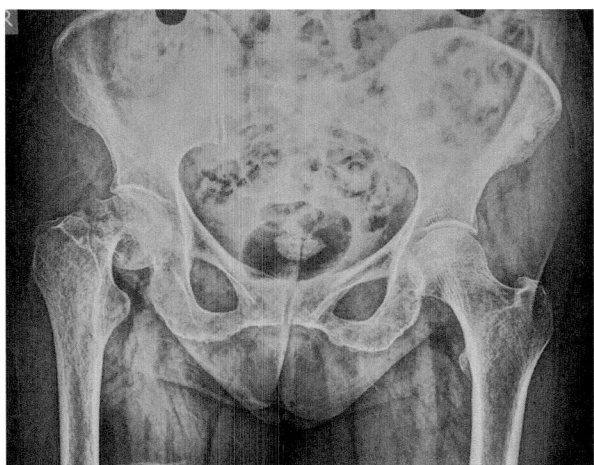

3.3   Intertrochanteric Fractures

Intertrochanteric fractures account for roughly half of all proximal femur fractures. An AP view of the pelvis is obtained, as well as a cross-table lateral view of the affected proximal femur. A physician-assisted internal rotation view of the fractured hip may be beneficial in further clarifying the fracture pattern (Figs. 3.4 and 3.5).

The **Boyd and Griffin classification** is based on the involvement of subtrochanteric region:

- **Type I**: linear intertrochanteric
- **Type II**: with comminution of trochanteric region
- **Type III**: with comminution associated with the subtrochanteric component
- **Type IV**: oblique fracture of the shaft with extension into the subtrochanteric region

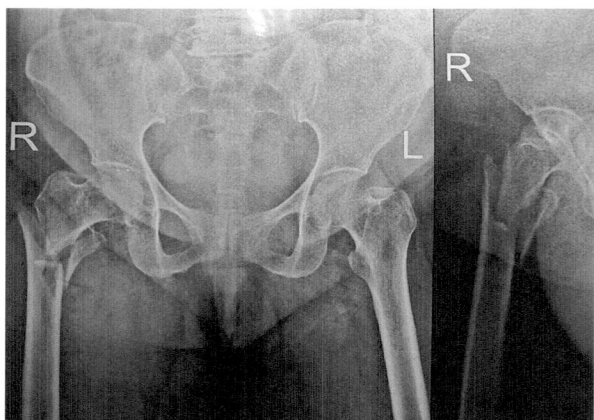

Fig. 3.4 X-ray pelvis with both hip AP and right hip lateral view showing intertrochanteric fracture

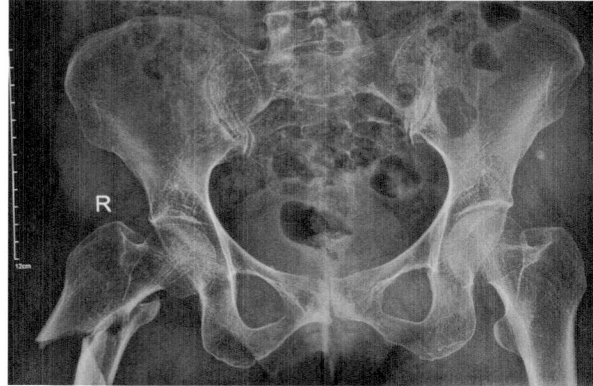

Fig. 3.5 X-ray pelvis with both hip AP view showing intertrochanteric fracture of right femur (reverse oblique type)

3.4   Subtrochanteric Fractures

Subtrochanteric fractures account for 10–30% of all hip fractures and can affect people of all ages. An AP view of the pelvis should be taken, as well as lateral views of the hip and femur. The entire femur, including the knee, should be evaluated (Fig. 3.6).

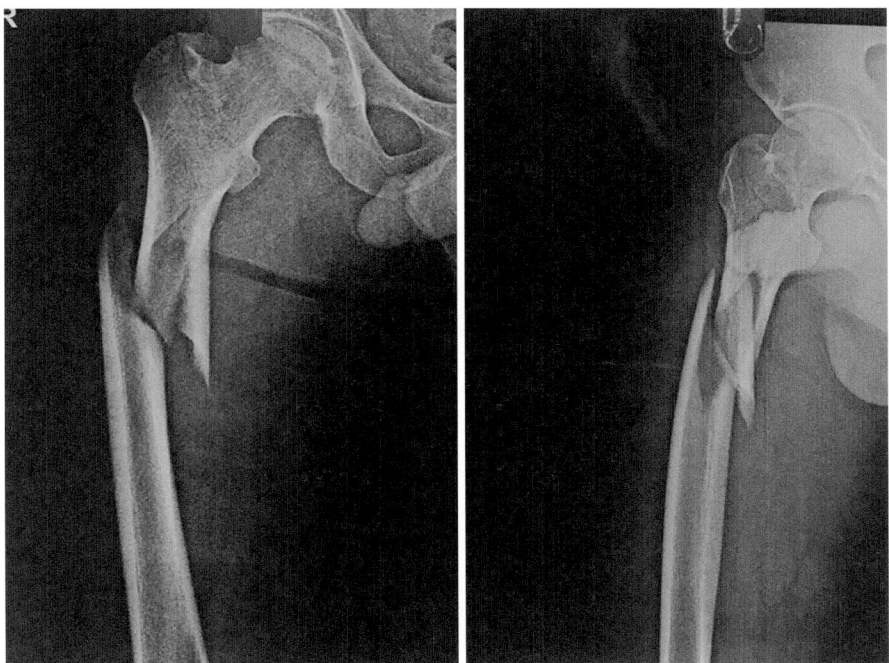

Fig. 3.6 X-ray of proximal femur AP and lateral view showing subtrochanteric fracture with butterfly fragment

3.5   Distal Femur Fractures

Fractures of the distal femur account for around 7% of all femur fractures. AP, lateral, and 45-degree oblique radiographs of the distal femur may be taken. The entire femur should be radiographically evaluated. Traction views can assist in assessing the fracture pattern and intra-articular extension more accurately. Contralateral views can help with comparison and can also be used as a template for preoperative planning (Figs. 3.7 and 3.8).

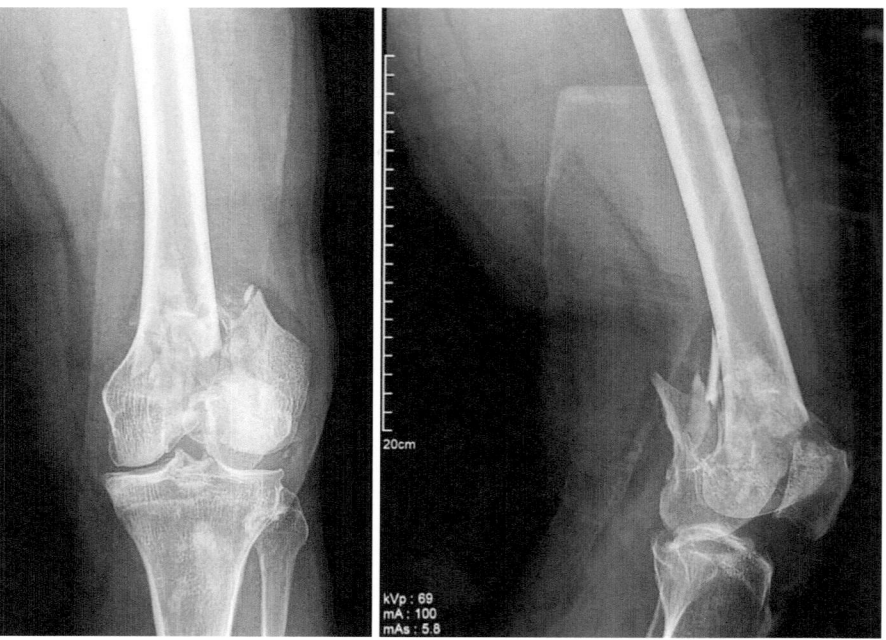

Fig. 3.7 AP and lateral view of knee showing intercondylar fracture of distal femur

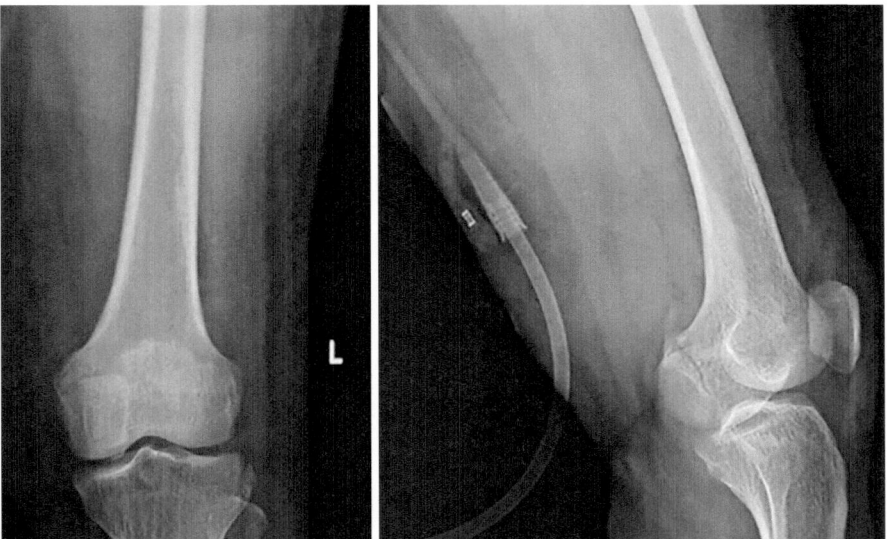

Fig. 3.8 AP and lateral view of knee showing fracture of lateral condyle of femur in the coronal plane (Hoffa's fracture)

3.6   Knee Dislocation

Traumatic knee dislocation is a rare but potentially life-threatening condition that should be treated as an orthopaedic emergency. Because neurovascular injury is so common, urgent reduction is advised before radiographic examination.

Anteroposterior (AP) and lateral images of the knee should be acquired following the reduction to assess the reduction and identify any associated injuries. Soft tissue interposition and the necessity for open reduction may be indicated by widened knee joint gaps. Findings on X-Ray: Obvious dislocation, Irregular/asymmetric joint space, Lateral capsular sign, Avulsion, Osteochondral defects (Fig. 3.9).

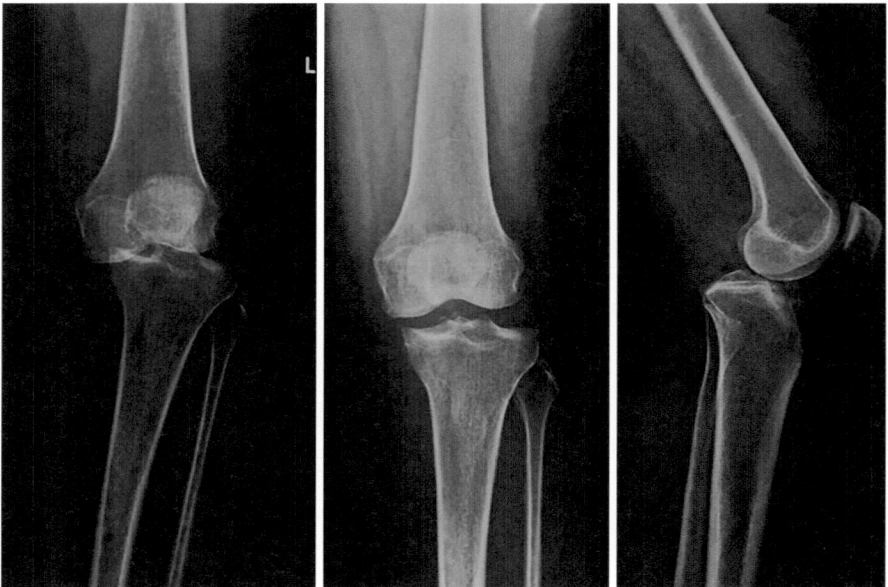

Fig. 3.9   X-ray showing posterior dislocation of knee

3.7   Patella Fracture

The AP and lateral X-rays of the knee should be taken. A bipartite patella can be mistaken for a fracture; it usually occurs in the superolateral position and has smooth borders; it is bilateral in 50% of cases. Displaced fractures are frequently visible on lateral view. An axial view (sunrise) may aid in the detection of osteochondral or vertical marginal fractures. In acute setting, this view may be difficult to obtain (Fig. 3.10).

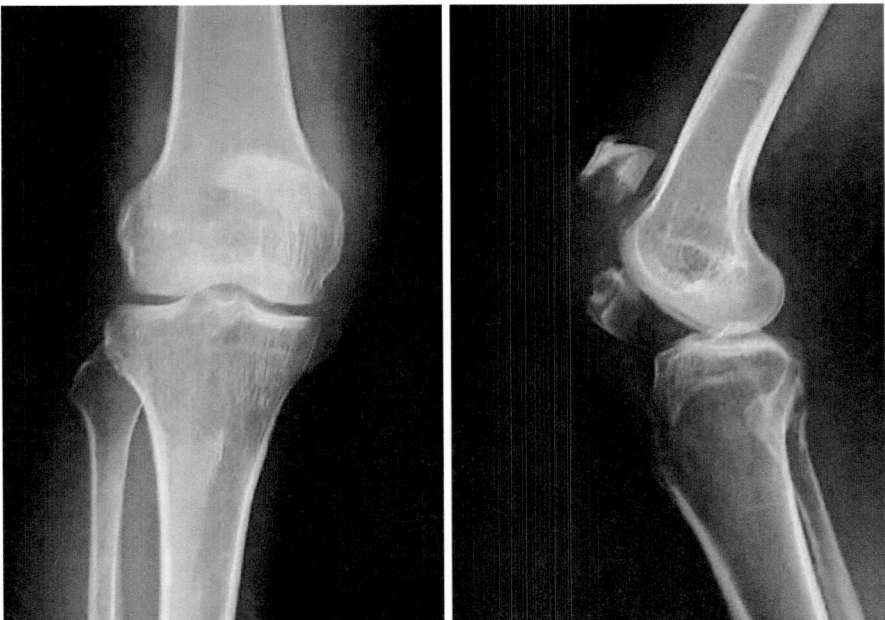

Fig. 3.10 AP and lateral view of knee showing transverse fracture of patella

3.8   Proximal Tibia Fractures

Tibial plateau fractures account for 1% of all fractures and 8% of fractures in the elderly population. Isolated lateral plateau fractures account for 55–70% of tibial plateau fractures, compared to 10–25% isolated medial plateau fractures and 10–30% bicondylar lesions.

AP and lateral views should be taken, as well as 40° internal (lateral plateau) and exterior (medial plateau) oblique projections. The Segond sign (lateral capsular avulsion) and the Pellegrini–Stieda lesion (calcification at the insertion of the medial collateral ligament noticed late) are all signs of concomitant ligamentous injury. In higher energy injuries with significant impaction and metadiaphyseal fragmentation, a physician-assisted traction view can aid to better define the fracture pattern and establish the efficacy of ligamentotaxis for fracture reduction.

3.9   Schatzker Classification

Type I: Lateral plateau, split fracture
Type II: Lateral plateau, split depression fracture (most common)
Type III: Lateral plateau, depression fracture
Type IV: Medial plateau fracture
Type V: Bicondylar plateau fracture
Type VI: Plateau fracture with separation of the metaphysis from the diaphysis (Fig. 3.11)

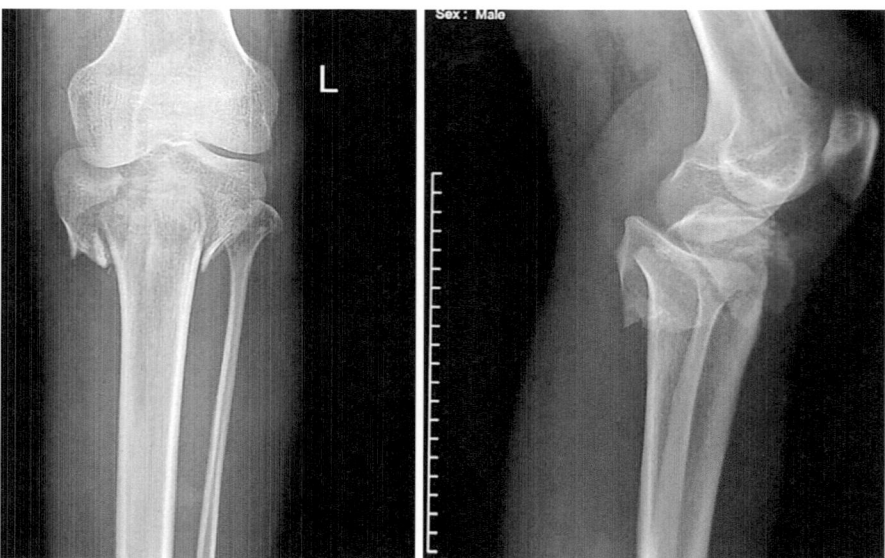

Fig. 3.11 AP and lateral radiograph of knee showing bicondylar fracture of proximal tibia with metaphysio-diaphyseal dissociation

3.10   Ankle Fractures

Isolated malleolar fractures account for two-thirds of all ankle fractures, with bimalleolar fractures accounting for a quarter of patients and trimalleolar fractures accounting for the remaining 5–10%.

Ankle AP, lateral, and mortise views should be taken. Tibiofibula overlap of 10 mm is abnormal and indicates syndesmotic injury in the AP view. A clear area of >5 mm between the tibia and fibula is abnormal and indicates syndesmotic damage. A discrepancy in breadth of more than 2 mm between the medial and lateral sides of the superior joint space is abnormal and implies medial or lateral disruption. Lateral view: The talus dome should be centred beneath the tibia and parallel to the tibial plafond. The direction of fibular injury, as well as posterior tibial tuberosity fractures, can be determined. The anterior capsule avulsion fractures of the talus can be detected. A syndesmotic injury is defined as anterior or posterior translation of the fibula in respect to the tibia in comparison to the unaffected side. Mortise view: The foot is rotated 15–20° internally to offset the intermalleolar axis. A lateral talar displacement is indicated by a medial clean gap more than 4–5 mm. The angle formed by the intermalleolar line and a line parallel to the articular surface of the distal tibia should be between 8 and 15°. The unaffected ankle's angle should be between 2 and 3°. Syndesmotic disruption is indicated by a 1 cm tibiofibular overlap. A talar displacement of more than 1 mm is considered abnormal (Fig. 3.12 and 3.13).

Fig. 3.12 AP and lateral radiograph of ankle showing bimalleolar fracture with ankle dislocation

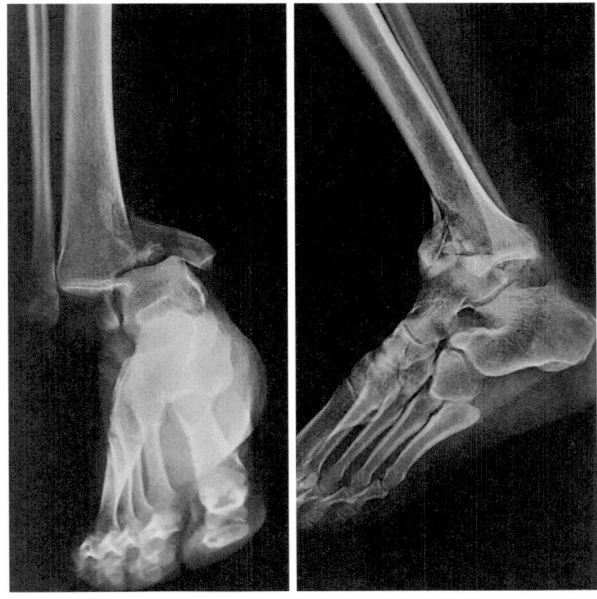

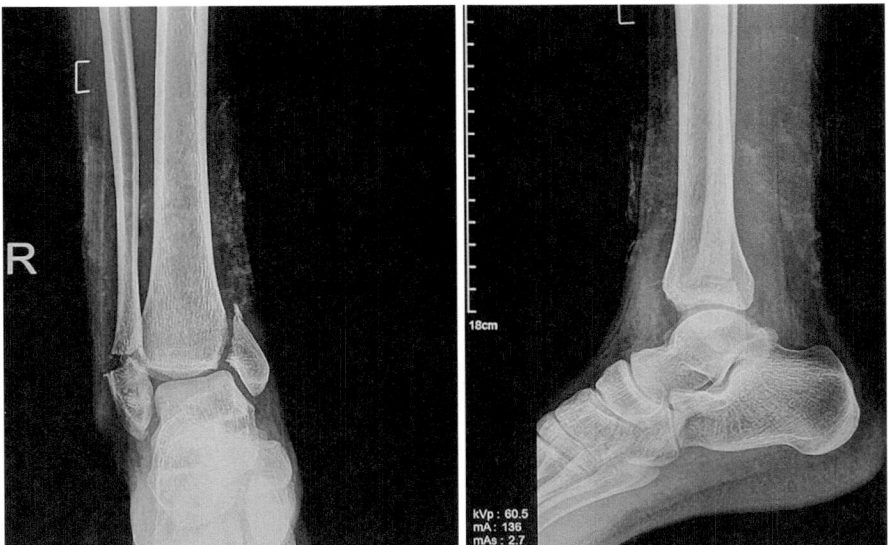

Fig. 3.13 AP and lateral radiograph of ankle showing bimalleolar fracture

3.11   Talus Fracture

Radiographs of the ankle (AP, lateral, and mortise), as well as AP, lateral, and oblique views of the foot, are obtained.

3.12   Hawkins Classification of Talar Neck Fractures

Type I: Nondisplaced
Type II: Associated subtalar subluxation or dislocation
Type III: Associated subtalar and ankle dislocation
Type IV: Type III with associated talonavicular subluxation or dislocation (Fig. 3.14)

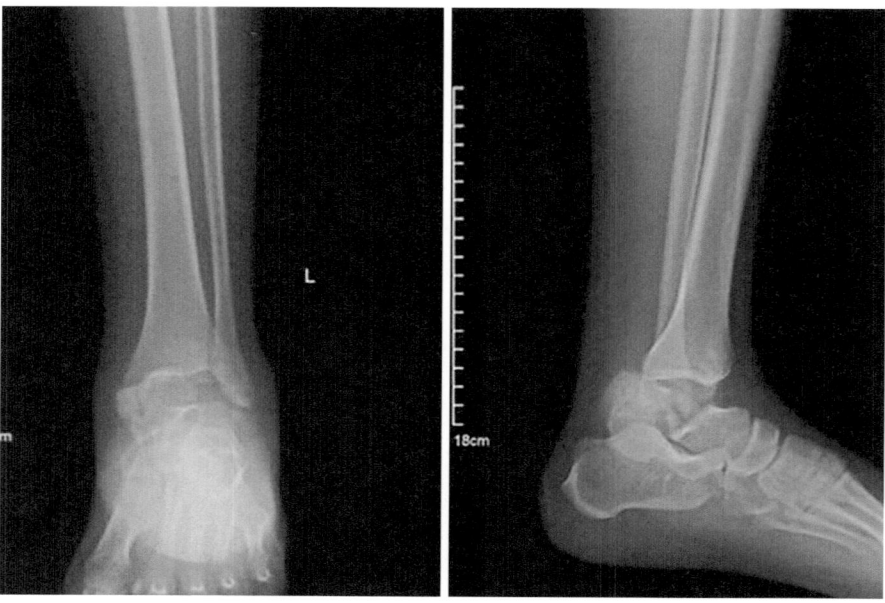

Fig. 3.14   AP and lateral view of ankle showing comminuted talar neck fracture (Hawkins Type 3)

3.13   Calcaneal Fractures

A lateral image of the hindfoot, an anteroposterior (AP) view of the foot, a Harris axial view, and an ankle series should be included in the initial radiographic evaluation of the patient with a suspected calcaneus fracture.

A line drawn tangentially from the posterior facet to the superior edge of the tuberosity and a line drawn from the highest point of the anterior process of the calcaneus to the highest point of the posterior facet make up the Böhler angle. The angle should be between 20 and 40°; if it decreases, it means the weight-bearing posterior aspect of the calcaneus has collapsed, moving body weight anteriorly. Two strong cortical struts extending laterally produce the Gissane (crucial) angle, one along the lateral boundary of the posterior facet and the other prior to the calcaneus beak. These cortical struts are visible right behind the lateral process of the talus and form an obtuse angle between 105 and 135°; an increase in this angle implies posterior facet collapse (Figs. 3.15 and 3.16).

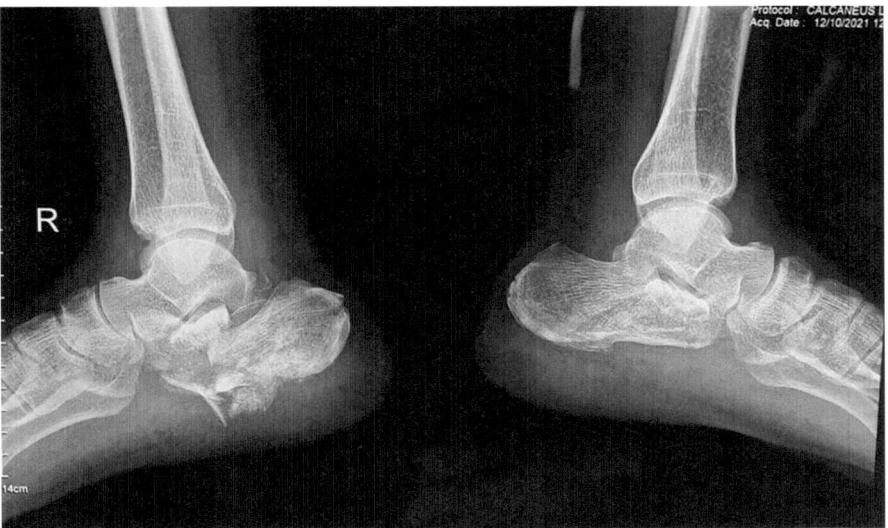

Fig. 3.15 Lateral view of calcaneum showing comminuted fracture of calcaneum

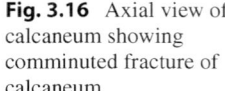

Fig. 3.16 Axial view of calcaneum showing comminuted fracture of calcaneum

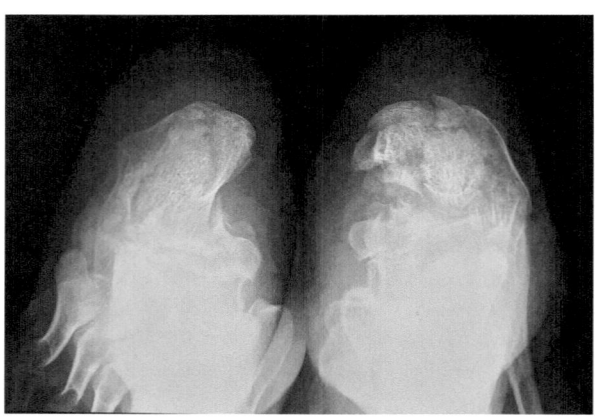

Bibliography

1. Egol KA Koval KJ Zuckerman JD Ovid Technologies Inc. *Handbook of Fractures*. Fifth ed. Philadelphia: Wolters Kluwer Health; 2015.
2. Greenspan A Beltran J. *Orthopedic Imaging : A Practical Approach*. Sixth ed. Philadelphia: Wolters Kluwer; 2015.

Radiography of Spine Trauma

4

Vertebral column fractures are important due to the structures affected as well as potential complications that could affect the spinal cord. Fractures of the vertebral column account for 3–6% of all skeletal injuries, and they most frequently affect adults between the ages of 20 and 50, with men accounting for 80% of all occurrences. The majority of spinal fractures happen at the thoracic and lumbar levels; however injuries to the cervical region have a higher risk of damaging the spinal cord. Typically, spinal injuries are caused by car accidents, sports-related activities, and falls from heights.

4.1 Cervical Spine Trauma

Because the patient is frequently unconscious, there are often accompanying injuries, and needless movement puts the cervical cord at danger of being damaged, radiographic examination of a patient with cervical spine trauma can be challenging and is typically confined to one or two projections. The lateral view is the most useful projection in these circumstances, and depending on the situation, it can be obtained either conventionally or with the patient supine. Injuries to the anterior and posterior arches of C1, the odontoid process, which is visible in profile, and the anterior atlantal-dens gap can all be observed on this projection, which is sufficient to show the majority of traumatic pathologies of the cervical spine. The intervertebral disc gaps and prevertebral soft tissues can be properly assessed, and the bodies and spinous processes of C2–7 are clearly visible. The atlanto-odontoid distance can be measured on the lateral radiograph, which is particularly useful for revealing potential instability at C1–2 since an increase in this distance of more than 3 mm implies atlantoaxial subluxation. The C7 vertebra must be seen on the lateral projection of the cervical spine since it is the injury location that is most frequently disregarded.

© The Author(s), under exclusive license to Springer Nature Singapore Pte
Ltd. 2023
N. S. Kushwaha, M. B. Abbas, *A Guide to Musculoskeletal Radiology*,
https://doi.org/10.1007/978-981-99-6155-9_4

4.2   Thoracolumbar Spine Trauma

To define the stability of different fractures, a useful method is to classify acute injuries to the thoracic and lumbar segments using the three-column spine. A localised paraspinal line bulge brought on by oedema and bleeding can be used to identify subtle thoracic vertebral fractures. Chance fracture, also referred to as a seat belt fracture, is a horizontal fracture of the lumbar vertebral body that extends into the lamina and spinous process. There are four different types of fracture dislocations of the thoracic and lumbar spine, which are unstable injuries: flexion-rotation injury, posteroanterior shear injury, anteroposterior shear damage, and flexion-distraction injury.

The thoracic and lumbar spines are examined from the anterior-posterior (AP) and lateral radiographs. A burst fracture is characterised by abnormal expansion of the interpedicular space, which indicates lateral displacement of vertebral body fragments. By comparing the height of the injured level with nearby uninjured vertebrae, it is possible to calculate the loss of vertebral body height. Using the Cobb method, sagittal plane alignment can be quantified. Radiographs of the chest and abdomen taken during the initial trauma assessment are insufficient for determining spinal column injuries (Figs. 4.1 and 4.2).

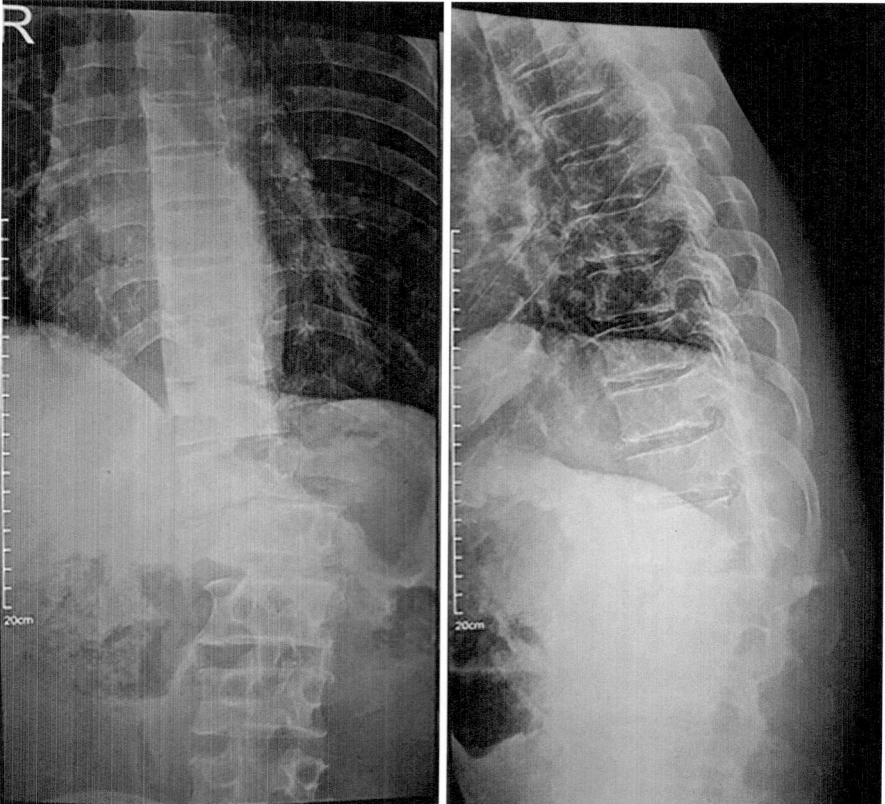

Fig. 4.1 AP and lateral view of dorso-lumbar spine showing fracture dislocation of L1 vertebrae

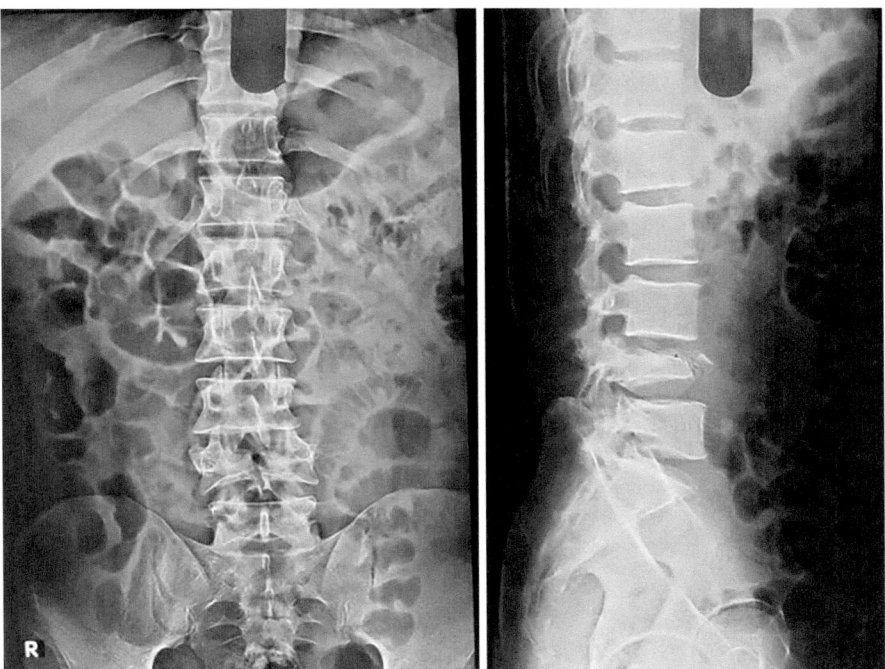

Fig. 4.2 AP and lateral view of lumbosacral spine showing wedge compression fracture of L4 vertebrae

Bibliography

1. Egol KA Koval KJ Zuckerman JD Ovid Technologies Inc. *Handbook of Fractures*. Fifth ed. Philadelphia: Wolters Kluwer Health; 2015.
2. Greenspan A Beltran J. *Orthopedic Imaging : A Practical Approach*. Sixth ed. Philadelphia: Wolters Kluwer; 2015.

Radiographs of Pelvi-acetabular and Sacroiliac Region

5

The majority of pelvic fractures in younger individuals are caused by high-energy trauma, whereas pelvic fractures in the elderly are caused by minor trauma, such as a fall.

Standard trauma radiographs include an AP view of the chest, a lateral view of the cervical spine, and an AP view of the pelvis. On AP of the pelvis, pubic rami fractures and symphysis displacement, sacroiliac joint and sacral fractures, iliac fractures, and L5 transverse process fractures can be visualised. The teardrop, the anterior wall, the posterior wall, the line illustrating the superior weight-bearing surface of the acetabulum, and the iliopectineal line (limit of anterior column) are all anatomic landmarks that should be visualised on AP radiograph. Iliac oblique radiograph (45° external rotation view): Posterior column (ilioischial line), the iliac wing, and the anterior wall of the acetabulum. Obturator oblique view (45° internal rotation view): Anterior column and posterior wall of the acetabulum. Inlet radiograph, taken with the patient supine with the tube directed 60° caudally, perpendicular to the pelvic brim, useful for determining anterior or posterior displacement of the sacroiliac joint, sacrum, or iliac wing. Outlet radiograph: This is taken with the patient supine with the tube directed 45° cephalad. Useful for determination of vertical displacement of the hemipelvis, may allow for visualisation of subtle signs of pelvic disruption, such as a slightly widened sacroiliac joint, discontinuity of the sacral borders, nondisplaced sacral fractures, or disruption of the sacral foramina (Figs. 5.1, 5.2, 5.3, 5.4, 5.5, and 5.6).

© The Author(s), under exclusive license to Springer Nature Singapore Pte Ltd. 2023
N. S. Kushwaha, M. B. Abbas, *A Guide to Musculoskeletal Radiology*,
https://doi.org/10.1007/978-981-99-6155-9_5

Fig. 5.1 Radiograph of pelvis with both hip AP view showing iliac blade fracture, with discontinuity in iliopubic and ilioischial line (both column acetabular fracture) with superior pubic ramus fracture

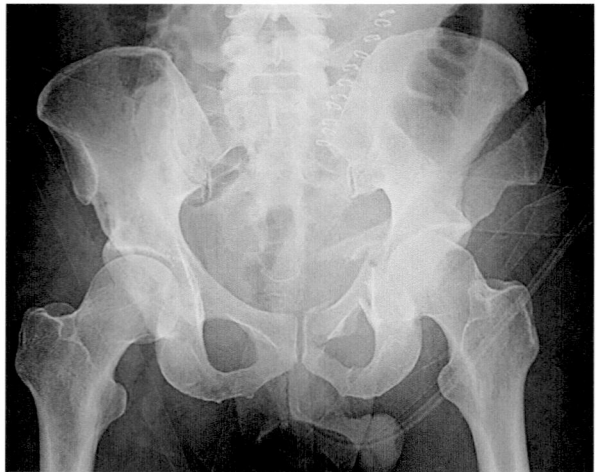

Fig. 5.2 Radiograph of pelvis with both hip AP view showing fracture of the acetabulum with migration of femoral head into the pelvis (central fracture dislocation)

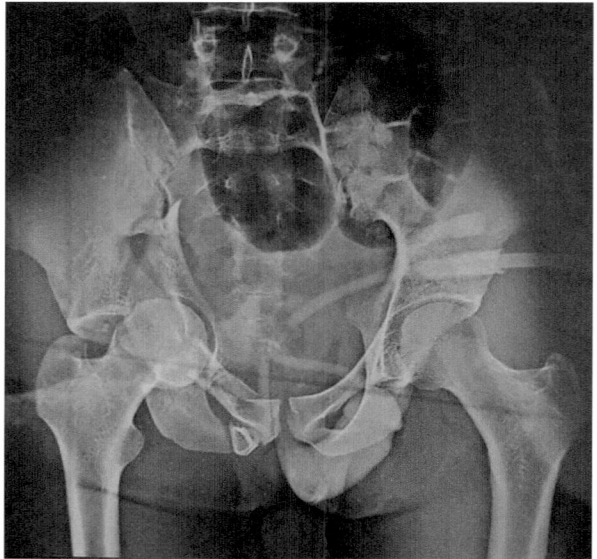

Fig. 5.3 Iliac oblique view of left hip showing break in iliopubic line with intact posterior column and anterior wall (anterior column fracture)

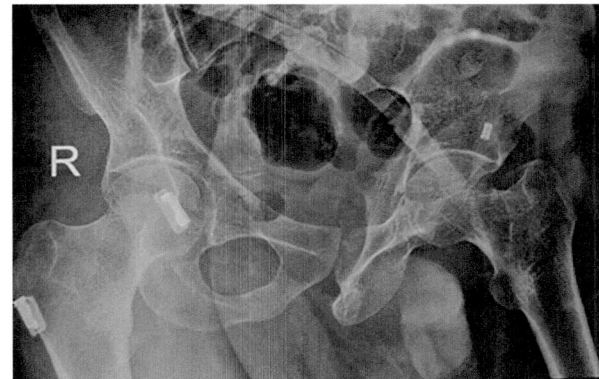

Fig. 5.4 Obturator oblique view of left hip showing break in iliopubic line and intact posterior wall (anterior column fracture)

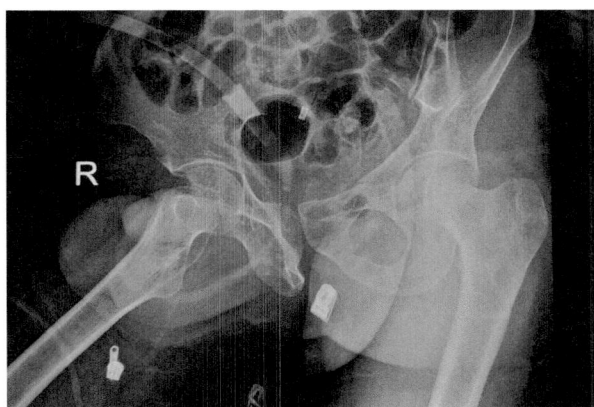

Fig. 5.5 Radiograph of pelvis with both hip AP view showing fracture of right superior and inferior pubic rami

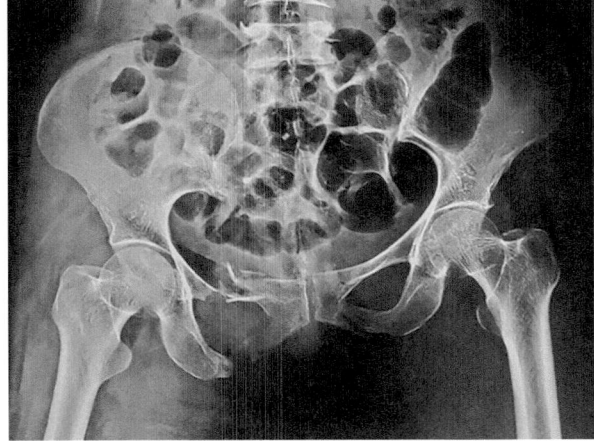

Fig. 5.6 Radiograph of pelvis with both hip AP view showing pubic diastasis with left sacroiliac joint disruption

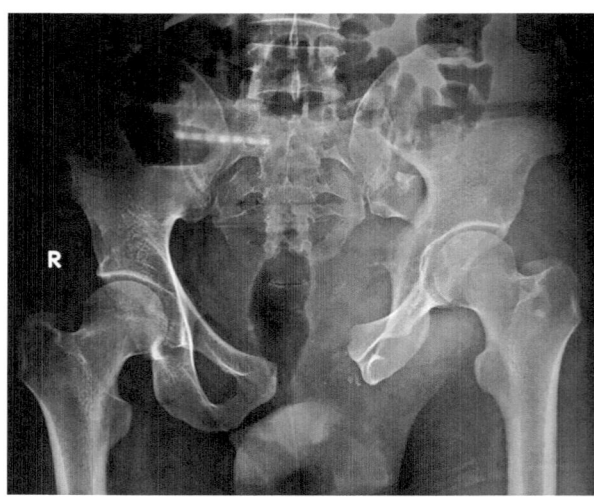

Bibliography

1. Egol KA Koval KJ Zuckerman JD Ovid Technologies Inc. *Handbook of Fractures*. Fifth ed. Philadelphia: Wolters Kluwer Health; 2015.
2. Greenspan A Beltran J. *Orthopedic Imaging : A Practical Approach*. Sixth ed. Philadelphia: Wolters Kluwer; 2015.

Radiographs of Paediatric Orthopaedic Trauma

6

Paediatric fractures are becoming more common. Increased sports activity has been blamed for the rise in fracture rates among youth. During their childhood, almost half of all children will fracture at least one bone. Skeletal trauma accounts for 10–15% of all childhood injuries, with physeal injuries accounting for 15–30% of these (phalanx fractures are the most common physeal injury).

Paediatric fractures occur at a lower energy than adult fractures due to structural variations. The majority of them are caused by compression, torsion, or bending moments. Compression fractures, often known as "buckle fractures" or "torus fractures", are most commonly observed near the metaphyseal diaphyseal junction. Torus fractures rarely result in physeal damage; however, they can induce acute angular deformity. Torus fractures are stable and rarely require manipulative reduction since they are affected. Depending on the maturity of the physis, torsion injuries occur in two different fracture patterns. The diaphyseal bone fails before the physis in a very young infant with a thick periosteum, resulting in a long spiral fracture. A physeal fracture occurs in the older child after a similar torsional injury. Bending moments in a young child can result in "greenstick fractures", which are incompletely shattered bones with a plastic deformation on the concave side. To get a sufficient reduction, the fracture may need to be completed. Bending moments can also cause microscopic fractures, which cause plastic deformation of the bone with no obvious fracture lines on normal radiographs; this can result in irreversible deformity. Bending moments cause transverse or short oblique fractures in older children. A little butterfly fragment may be detected on occasion, but because paediatric bone fails more easily in compression, a buckling of the cortex is more likely.

Radiographs of the affected bone, as well as the joint proximal and distal to the suspected location of injury, should be taken. The entire extremity may be placed on the radiographic plate if the site of the suspected injury is unknown. To properly interpret plain radiographs, a full grasp of normal ossification patterns is required. Views of the opposite extremity in comparison may help to appreciate subtle abnormalities or to locate a minimally displaced fracture. These should only be obtained if there is a doubt about the presence of a fracture observed on a radiograph of an injured extremity, not on a regular basis. "Soft signs", like the posterior fat pad indication in the elbow, should be carefully examined (Figs. 6.1, 6.2, 6.3, 6.4, and 6.5).

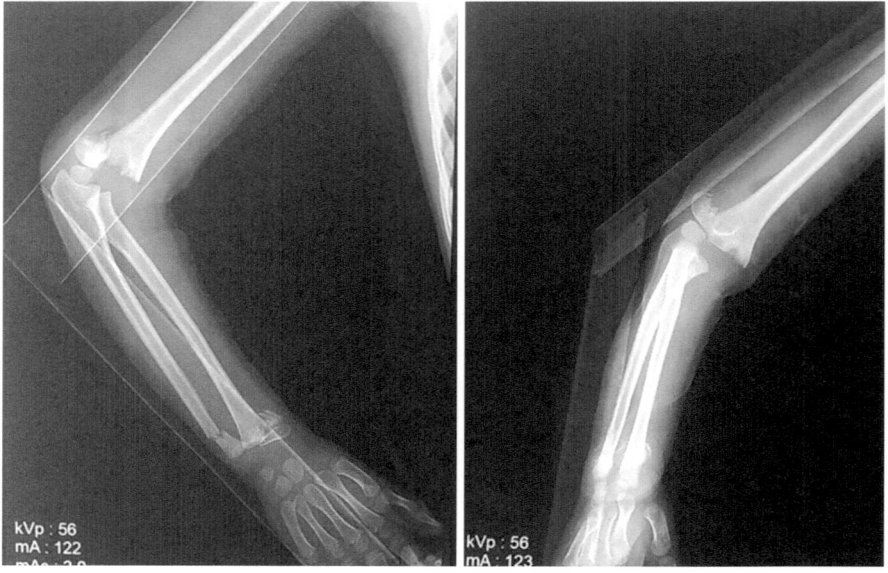

Fig. 6.1 X-ray of elbow showing supracondylar humerus fracture

Fig. 6.2 X-ray of wrist showing epiphyseal injury of distal end radius

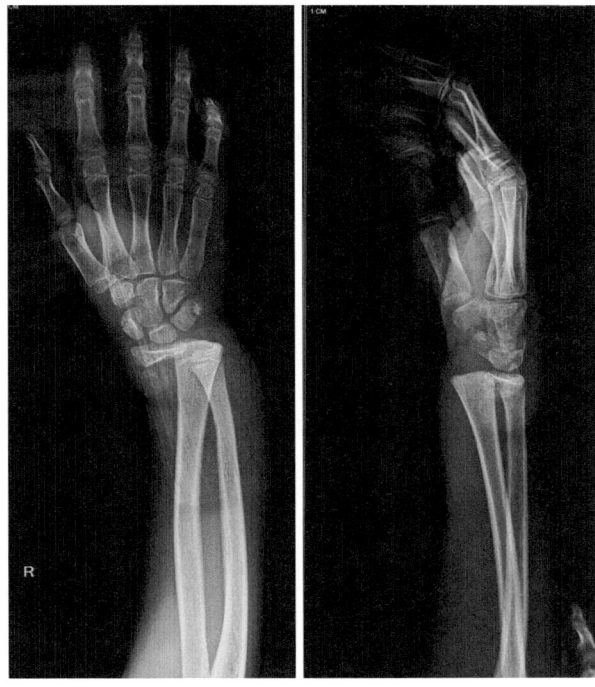

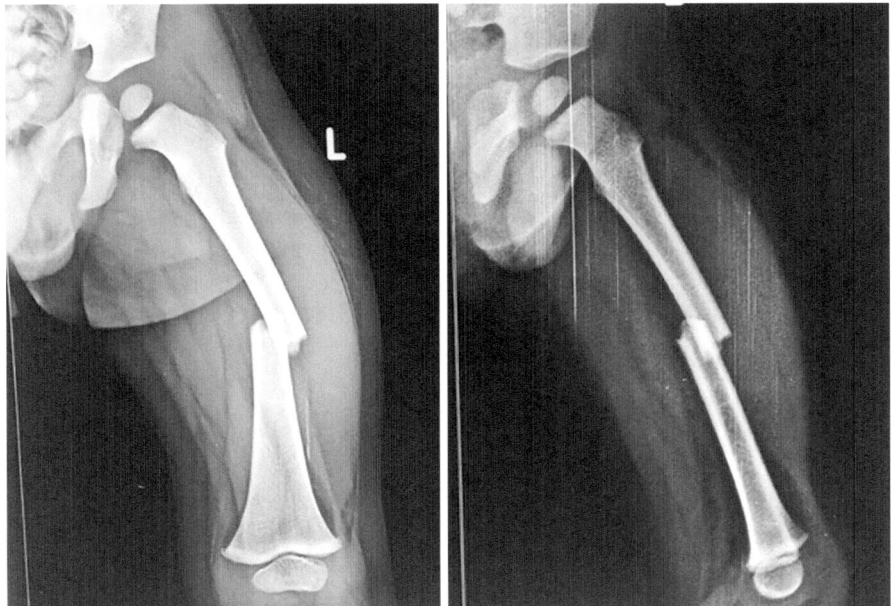

Fig. 6.3 X-ray of thigh showing fracture of mid-shaft of femur

Fig. 6.4 X-ray of leg
showing fracture of
mid-shaft of tibia and
fibula

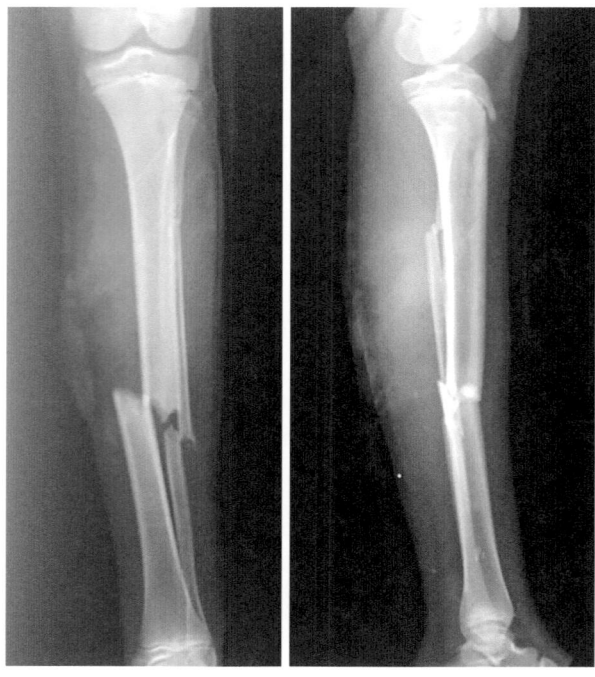

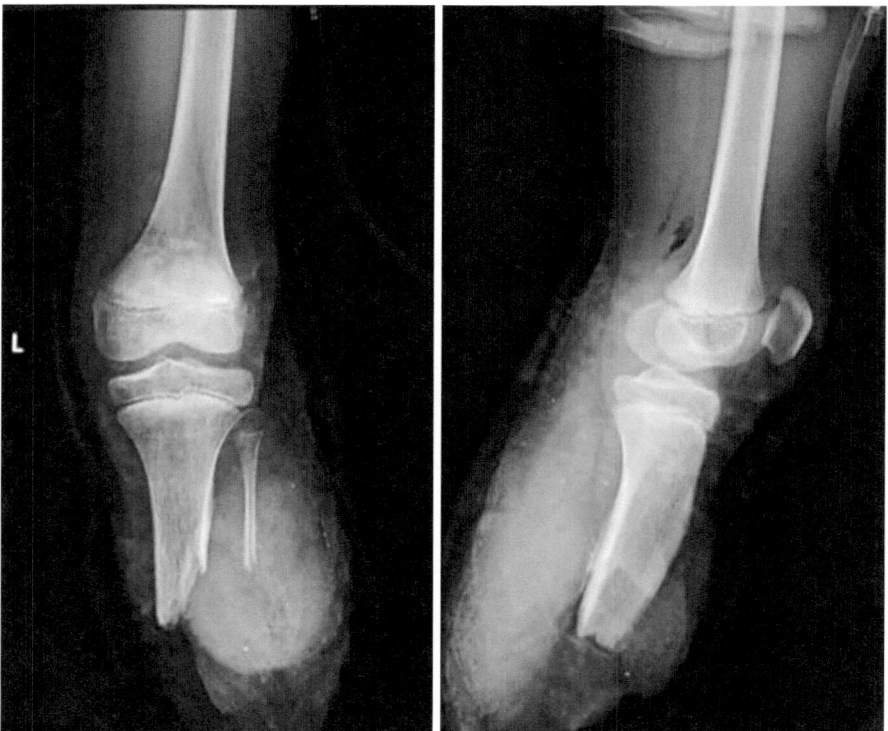

Fig. 6.5 X-ray showing traumatic amputation of proximal leg

Bibliography

1. Egol KA Koval KJ Zuckerman JD Ovid Technologies Inc. *Handbook of Fractures.* Fifth ed. Philadelphia: Wolters Kluwer Health; 2015.
2. Greenspan A Beltran J. *Orthopedic Imaging : A Practical Approach.* Sixth ed. Philadelphia: Wolters Kluwer; 2015.
3. Cepela DJ, Tartaglione JP, Dooley TP, Patel PN. Classifications In Brief: Salter-Harris Classification of Pediatric Physeal Fractures. Clin Orthop Relat Res. 2016 Nov;474(11):2531–2537. doi: 10.1007/s11999-016-4891-3. Epub 2016 May 20. PMID: 27206505; PMCID: PMC5052189.

Part III

Orthopaedic Oncology

Radiography in Orthopaedic Oncology

7

Bone tumours can be benign or malignant. Malignant tumours can be subclassified as primary, secondary, or metastatic (Table 7.1).

Description of a bony lesion/tumour
(a) Location/site of lesion (diaphyseal, metaphyseal, or epiphyseal)
(b) Border of the lesion (zone of transition, narrow/wide)
(c) Tumour matrix (osteoblastic, lytic, calcifications)
(d) Type of bone destruction (geographic, moth eaten, permeative)
(e) Periosteal reaction
(f) Soft tissue extension
(g) Number of lesions

© The Author(s), under exclusive license to Springer Nature Singapore Pte
Ltd. 2023
N. S. Kushwaha, M. B. Abbas, *A Guide to Musculoskeletal Radiology*,
https://doi.org/10.1007/978-981-99-6155-9_7

Table 7.1 Classification of tumours and tumour-like lesion by tissue of origin

Tissue of origin	Benign	Malignant
Bone forming (osteogenic)	Osteoma	Osteosarcoma
	Osteoid osteoma	
	Osteoblastoma	
Cartilage forming (chondrogenic)	Enchondroma	Chondrosarcoma
	Osteochondroma	
	Chondroblastoma	
	Chondromyxoid fibroma	
Fibrous, osteofibrous, and fibrocystic	Fibrous cortical defect	Fibrosarcoma
	Nonossifying fibroma	Malignant fibrous histiocytoma
	Fibrous dysplasia	
	Fibrocartilaginous dysplasia	
	Osteofibrous dysplasia	
Vascular	Haemangioma	Angiosarcoma
	Glomus tumour	Haemangioendothelioma
		Haemangiopericytoma
Haematopoietic, reticuloendothelial, and lymphatic	Giant cell tumour	Malignant giant cell tumour
	Langerhans cell histiocytosis	Lymphoma
	Lymphangioma	Leukaemia
		Myeloma
		Ewing's sarcoma
Neurogenic	Neurofibroma	Malignant Schwannoma
	Neurilemoma	Neuroblastoma
	Morton's neuroma	Primitive neuroectodermal tumour
		Chordoma
Notochordal, fat, and unknown	Lipoma	Liposarcoma
	Simple bone cyst	Adamantinoma
	Aneurysmal bone cyst	
	Intraosseous ganglion	

7.1   Benign Primary Bone Tumours

7.1.1   Osteoid Osteoma

A benign osteoblastic lesion defined by a nidus of osteoid tissue that may be entirely radiolucent or have a sclerotic core. The nidus has a limited growth capacity, measuring less than 1 cm in diameter most of the time. It is frequently surrounded by a reactive bone growth zone. The long bones, particularly the femur and tibia, are predisposed to these diseases in the young, mainly between the ages of 10 and 35 years.

7.1.2   Giant Cell Tumour

GCT of bone, also known as osteoclastoma, is an aggressive lesion with densely vascularised tissue, growing mononuclear stromal cells, and numerous uniformly distributed giant osteoclast cells. It is the sixth most frequent primary osseous neoplasm, accounting for around 5–8.6% of all primary bone tumours and approximately 23% of benign bone tumours. Long bones account for 60% of these lesions, with nearly all of them affecting the articular end of the bone. The proximal tibia, distal femur, distal radius, and proximal humerus are all good places to start. GCTs appear nearly exclusively when the growth plate has been erased, which occurs at skeletal maturity. The majority of patients are between the ages of 20 and 40, with a 2:1 female predominance.

GCT has distinct imaging characteristics. It is a radiolucent, primarily osteolytic lesion with a narrow zone of transition and no sclerotic margins, demonstrating geographic bone destruction and usually no periosteal reaction (Figs. 7.1 and 7.2).

7.1.3   Osteochondroma

Osteochondroma is a cartilage-capped bony outgrowth on the external surface of a bone, also known as osteocartilaginous exostosis. It is the most common benign

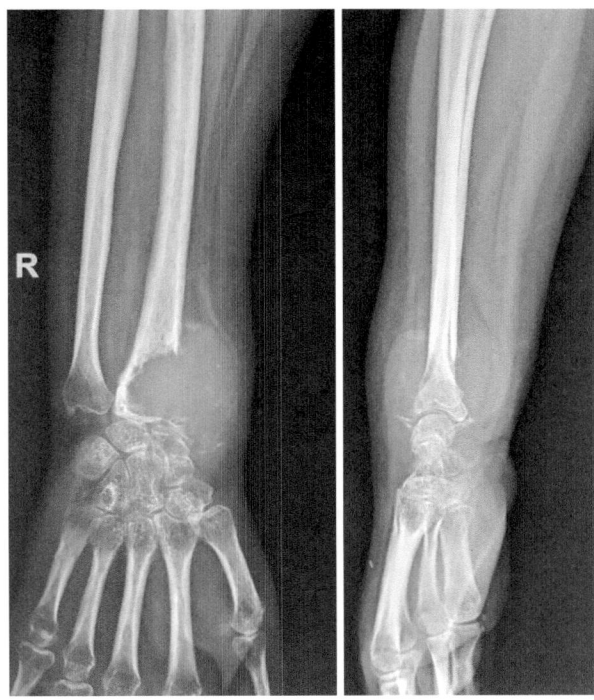

Fig. 7.1 AP and lateral radiograph of wrist showing well-defined osteolytic lesion in the distal end of radius with eccentric location, cortical breach, and soft tissue extension suggestive of GCT

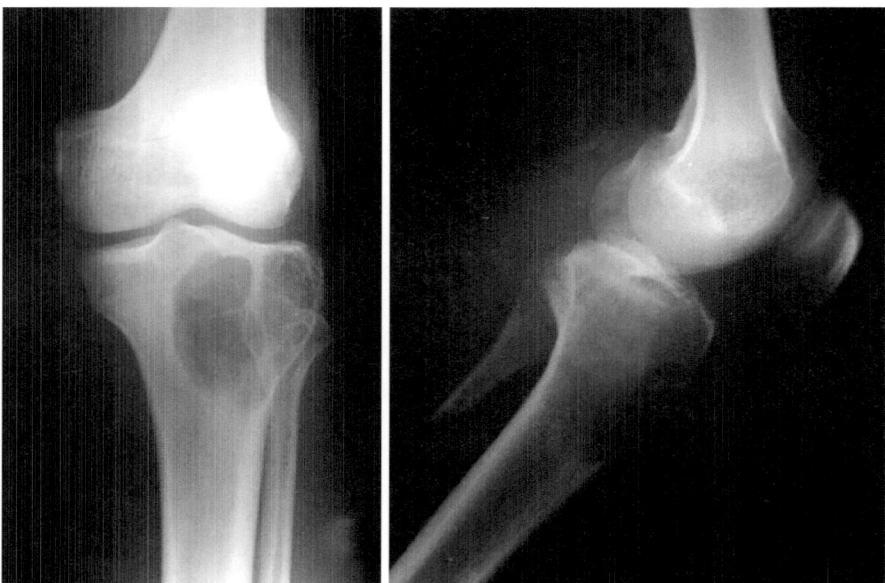

Fig. 7.2 AP and lateral radiograph of knee joint showing a purely osteolytic lesion in the proximal end of the tibia. Note its eccentric location, the absence of reactive sclerosis, and the extension of the lesion into the articular end of the bone, all characteristic features of GCT

bone lesion, accounting for between 20 and 50% of all benign bone tumours, and is usually identified before the third decade of life. At skeletal maturity, osteochondroma, which has its own growth plate, ceases growing. The metaphyses of the long bones, especially those at the knee and the proximal humerus, are the most typical sites of involvement.

The radiographic appearance of osteochondroma depends on whether the lesion is pedunculated, with a slender pedicle pointing out from the surrounding growth plate, or sessile, with a broad base linked to the cortex. The main distinguishing feature of either type of lesion is the continuous merging of the host bone's cortex with the cortex of the osteochondroma; also, the medullary component of the lesion and the nearby bone's medullary cavity are connected (Figs. 7.3 and 7.4).

7.1.4   Enchondroma

Enchondroma is the second most common benign bone tumour, accounting for about 10% of all benign bone tumours and being the most prevalent tumour of the hand's short tubular bones. An enchondroma is a lesion that is located centrally in

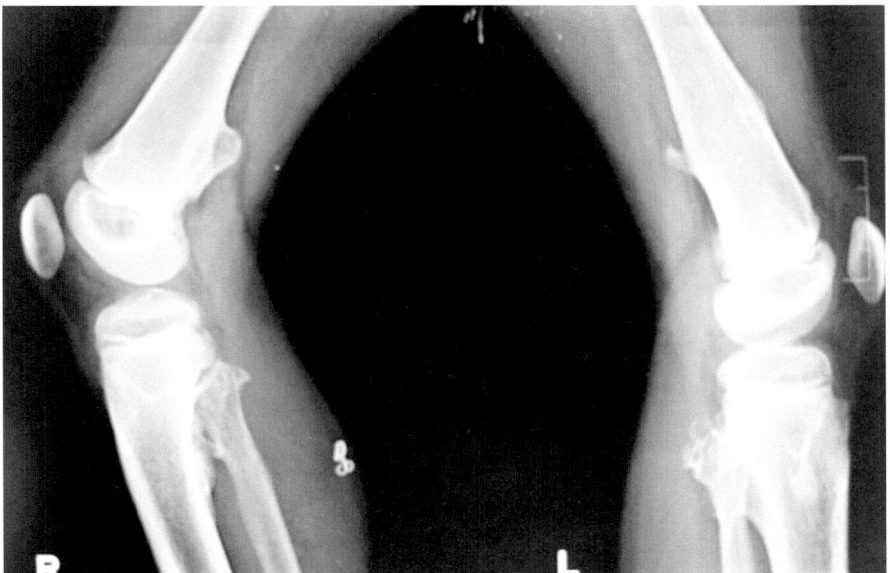

Fig. 7.3 AP and lateral radiograph of knee joint showing multiple bony outgrowths from distal end of femur and proximal end of tibia suggestive of osteochondroma

the bone; a chondroma is a lesion that is located extracortically (periosteally) (periosteal or juxtacortical). The growth of mature hyaline cartilage characterises this benign lesion, regardless of its location.

In most cases, radiography is sufficient to show the lesion. The lesion is generally completely radiolucent in short bones, although it may have obvious calcifications in long bones. Enchondromas are referred to as calcifying when the calcifications are widespread. Because cartilage grows in a lobular pattern, the lesions can also be identified by shallow scalloping of the inner (endosteal) cortical edges (Fig. 7.5).

7.1.5 Chondroblastoma

Chondroblastoma, also known as a Codman tumour, is a benign lesion that develops before skeletal maturity and typically affects the epiphyses of long bones like the humerus, tibia, and femur. It accounts for less than 1% of all primary bone cancers. Although secondary metaphysis involvement beyond skeletal maturity has been documented, a primarily metaphyseal or diaphyseal location is extremely uncommon.

Fig. 7.4 AP radiograph of
knee joint showing
pedunculated bony
outgrowth from the distal
end of femur suggestive of
osteochondroma

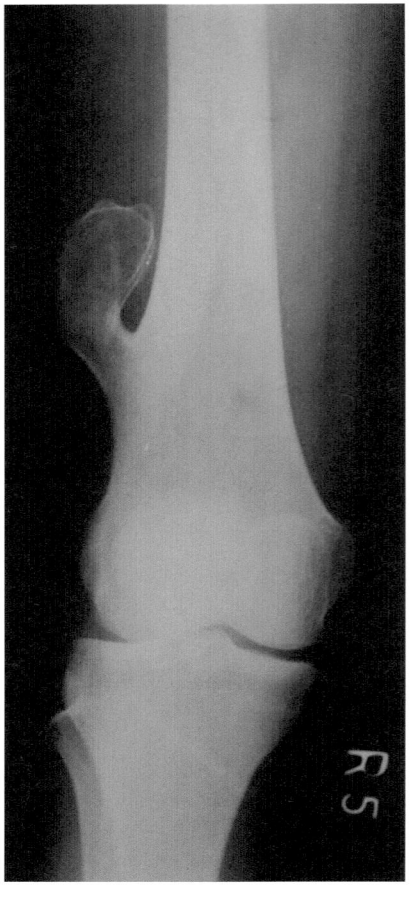

Although the lesion is most commonly found in growing bones, it has been reported in cases where the growth plate has been obliterated. Chondroblastoma is frequently seen eccentrically, has a sclerotic border, and exhibits sporadic matrix calcifications (25% of cases) (Fig. 7.6).

7.1.6   Fibrous Cortical Defect and Nonossifying Fibroma

The most frequent fibrous lesions of bone are fibrous cortical defects and nonossifying (nonosteogenic) fibromas, which are mostly observed in children and adolescents. They occur in long bones, notably the femur and tibia, and are more common in boys than in girls.

Asymptomatic fibrous cortical defect is prevalent in 30% of normal people in their first and second decades of life. The elliptical radiolucent lesion is restricted

Fig. 7.5 Radiograph shows radiolucent lesion in middle phalanx of third finger with pathological fracture suggestive of enchondroma

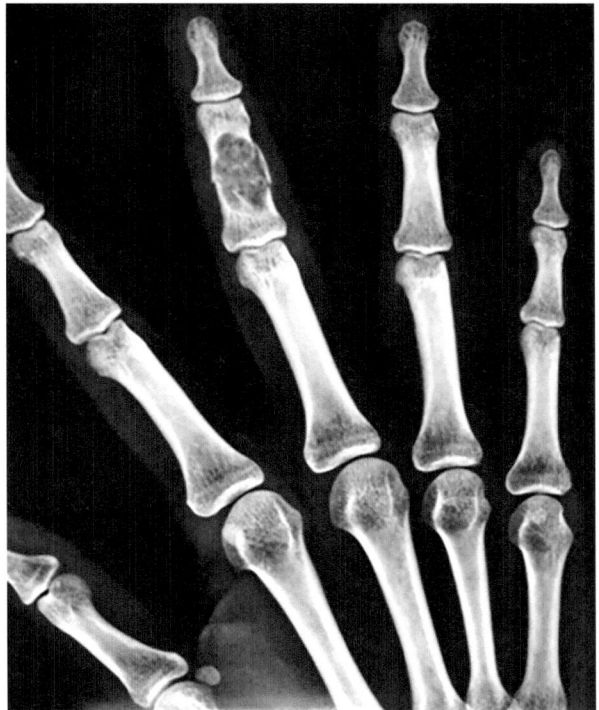

to the cortex of a long bone near the growth plate and is defined by a thin sclerotic margin. The majority of these lesions will go away on their own, but a few may continue to grow. They are called nonossifying fibroma when they encroach on the medullary area of a bone. These lesions, which are often positioned eccentrically in the bone, develop a scalloped sclerotic border with continuous growth.

7.1.7   Fibrous Dysplasia

Fibrous dysplasia can affect a single bone (monostotic) or multiple bones (polyostotic). It is defined by the replacement of normal lamellar cancellous bone with an aberrant fibrous tissue containing tiny, irregularly organised trabeculae of immature woven bone formed by fibrous stromal metaplasia.

The proportion of osseous-to-fibrous composition affects the radiographic appearance of fibrous dysplasia. Lesions with more osseous composition are denser and sclerotic, whereas those with more fibrous substance are more radiolucent and have a distinctive groundglass appearance.

Fig. 7.6 AP view of knee joint showing well-defined radiolucent lesion in the distal epiphysis of femur suggestive of chondroblastoma

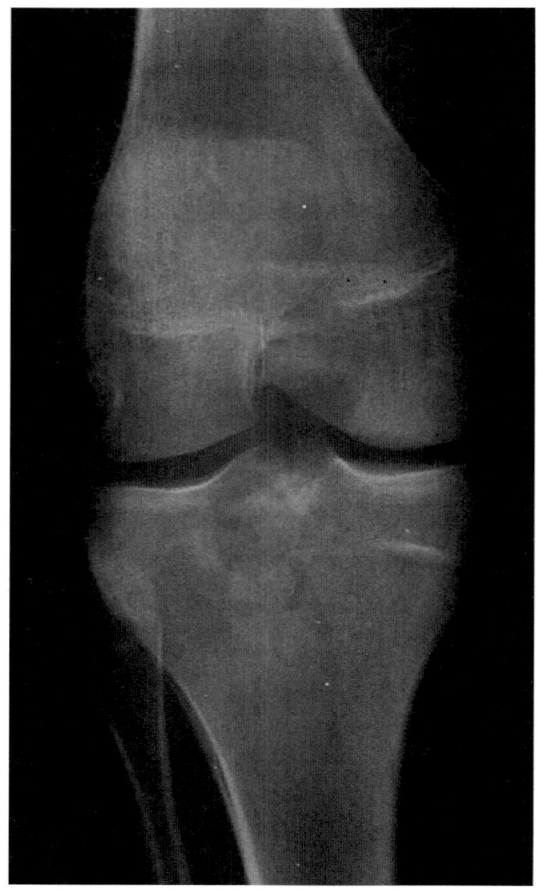

7.1.8 Simple Bone Cyst

The simple bone cyst (SBC), also known as a unicameral bone cyst, is a tumour-like lesion with an unexplained aetiology that accounts for about 3% of all primary bone lesions. It is thought to be caused by a localised disruption of bone development. SBC appears to be reactive or developing rather than a true neoplasm, despite the fact that the pathophysiology is still unknown. It is more common in boys than girls and usually appears in the first two decades of life. SBCs are most commonly found in the proximal diaphysis of the humerus and femur, particularly in skeletally immature patients.

The first sign of the lesion is generally a pathologic fracture. SBC presents as a radiolucent, centrally placed, well-circumscribed lesion with sclerotic edges on radiography. There is no periosteal reaction, which distinguishes an SBC from an aneurysmal bone cyst (ABC), which always has some periosteal response; nevertheless, there is periosteal reactivity in the case of pathologic fracture (Fig. 7.7).

Fig. 7.7 AP radiograph of humerus showing well-defined radiolucent lesion in the proximal humerus with pathological fracture in a skeletally immature patient suggestive of simple bone cyst

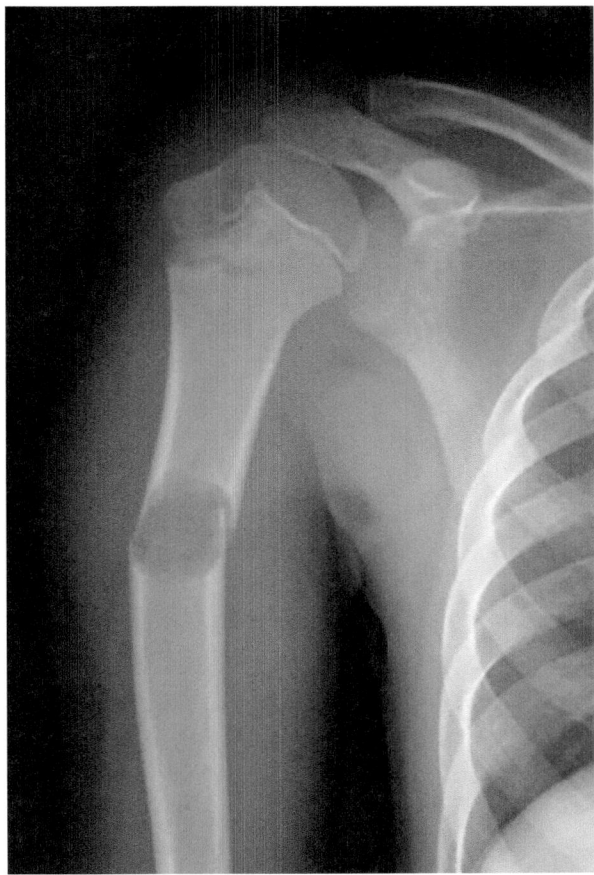

7.1.9   Aneurysmal Bone Cyst

ABC accounts for roughly 6% of all primary bone lesions and is most commonly found in children; 90% of these lesions occur in patients under the age of 20. ABCs are most commonly found in the metaphysis of long bones, but they can also be found in the diaphysis of long bones, flat bones like the scapula or pelvis, and even the vertebrae. These lesions can arise spontaneously or as a result of cystic alterations in an existing lesion like a chondroblastoma, osteoblastoma, giant cell tumour (GCT), or fibrous dysplasia. Multicystic eccentric expansion of the bone with a buttress or thin shell of periosteal reaction is the radiographic hallmark of an ABC (Fig. 7.8).

Fig. 7.8 AP and lateral
view of distal leg showing
expansile radiolucent
lesion in the distal
metaphysis of tibia with
multiple septations
suggestive of ABC

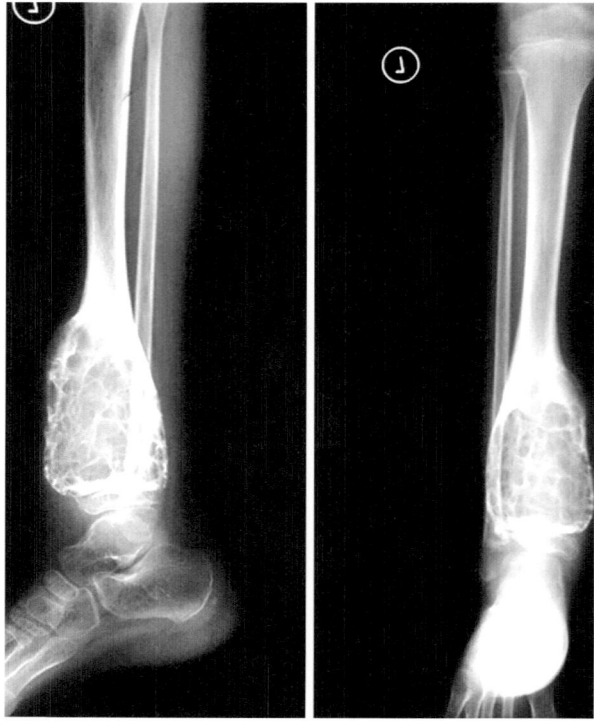

Bibliography

1. Greenspan A Beltran J. *Orthopedic Imaging : A Practical Approach*. Sixth ed. Philadelphia: Wolters Kluwer; 2015.
2. Picci P, Manfrini M, Fabbri N, et al., editors. Atlas of musculoskeletal tumors and tumorlike lesions: the Rizzolo case archive. Cham: Springer; 2020.
3. Yochum TR Rowe LJ. *Yochum and Rowe's Essentials of Skeletal Radiology*. 3rd ed. Philadelphia: Lippincott/Williams & Wilkins; 2005.

Radiographs of Malignant Primary Bone Tumours

8

8.1 Osteosarcoma

Osteosarcoma (osteogenic sarcoma) is a type of primary malignant bone tumour that accounts for about 20% of all primary bone malignancies. There are different forms of osteosarcoma, each with its own clinical, imaging, and histologic features. The osteoid and bone matrix are formed by malignant connective tissue cells, which is a common trait of all types. It can be primary, secondary, extra-skeletal, or metastatic.

Medullary and cortical bone destruction, an aggressive periosteal reaction, a soft tissue mass, and tumour bone either within the destructive lesion or at its periphery, as well as within the soft tissue mass, are all radiologic hallmarks of conventional osteosarcoma. The type of bone loss may not be apparent on conventional studies in some cases, but uneven densities suggesting tumour bone and an aggressive periosteal reaction are diagnostic indicators. The amount of tumour bone formation, calcified matrix, and osteoid determine the degree of radiopacity in the tumour. Tumours can appear as solely sclerotic or strictly osteolytic lesions, but they usually combine the two. The borders are frequently blurry, with a large transition zone. Moth-eaten or permeative bone destruction is the most common, whereas geographic bone destruction is unusual. The "sunburst" type of periosteal reaction and a Codman triangle are the most frequent types of periosteal reaction seen with osteosarcoma; the lamellated (onion skin) type of reaction is less common (Figs. 8.1 and 8.2).

N. S. Kushwaha, M. B. Abbas, *A Guide to Musculoskeletal Radiology*, https://doi.org/10.1007/978-981-99-6155-9_8

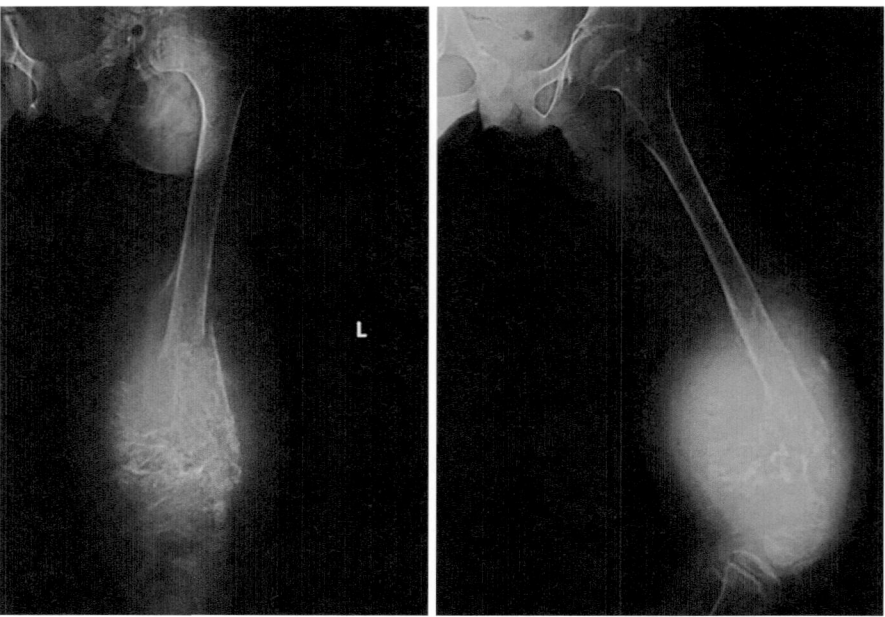

Fig. 8.1 AP and lateral radiograph of skeletally immature patient showing typical medullary and cortical bone destruction in the distal metaphysis of femur with pathological fracture with sunburst periosteal reaction and soft tissue invasion

Fig. 8.2 Lateral radiograph of distal metaphyseal end of femur showing cortical and medullary bone destruction with sunburst periosteal reaction and tumour bone formation with soft tissue invasion

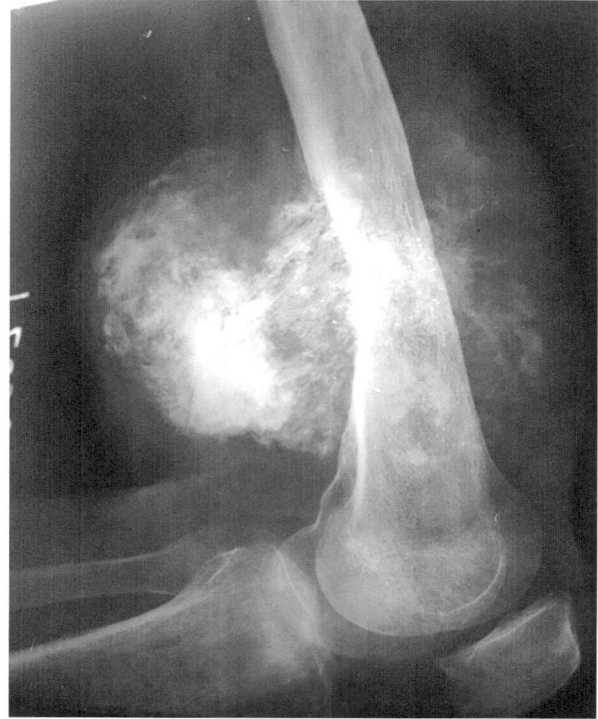

8.2   Chondrosarcoma

Chondrosarcoma is a type of malignant bone tumour in which tumour cells produce a cartilage matrix. Males have double the chances as females to have chondrosarcoma. Adults, particularly those in their third decade, are more likely to develop. The pelvic and long bones, especially the femur and humerus, are the most common places. The majority of chondrosarcomas are slow-growing tumours that are commonly found by chance. Can be primary, secondary, or metastatic.

On radiographs, a typical chondrosarcoma appears as an expansile lesion in the medulla, with thickening of the cortex and deep endosteal scalloping; popcorn-like, annular, or comma-shaped calcifications are visible in the medullary part of the bone (Fig. 8.3).

Fig. 8.3 Radiograph of pelvis with both hip AP view showing large calcified mass arising from right pelvic bone suggestive of chondrosarcoma

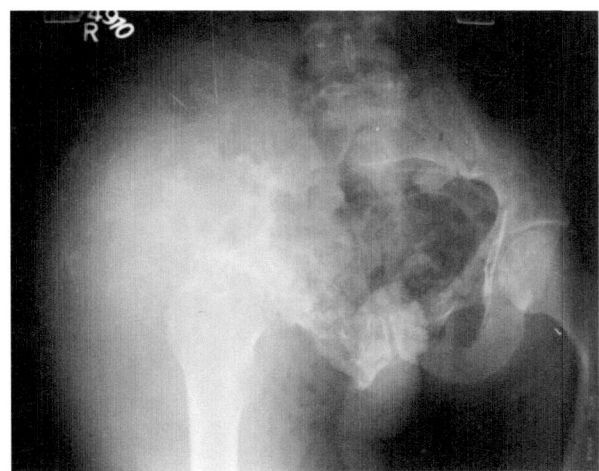

8.3   Ewing Sarcoma

Ewing sarcoma is a highly aggressive neoplasm that primarily affects children and adolescents with a strong male preponderance. Ewing sarcoma is considered to arise from bone marrow cells; however the exact histogenesis is uncertain.

The diaphysis of the long bones, as well as the ribs and flat bones like the scapula and pelvis, is particularly prone to Ewing sarcoma. The lesion is poorly defined, with permeative or moth-eaten bone degradation and a massive soft tissue mass, as well as an aggressive periosteal response with an onion skin (or "onion peel") or, less typically, a "sunburst" look (Fig. 8.4).

Fig. 8.4 AP radiograph of humerus showing a radiolucent lesion in the diaphyseal region with wide zone of transition with pathological fracture suggestive of Ewing sarcoma

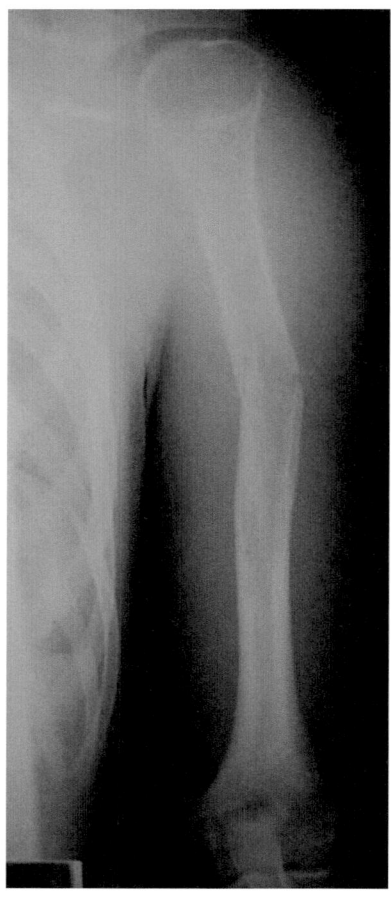

8.4   Multiple Myeloma

Multiple myeloma is the most common primary malignant bone tumour. It starts in the bone marrow. It is responsible for 10% of all haematologic malignancies and 1% of all cancers. It occurs more frequently in men than in women between the fifth and seventh decades. Although the axial skeleton (head, spine, ribs, and pelvis) is the most usually affected area, any bone can be involved.

It usually has multiple lytic lesions dispersed throughout the skeleton. The skull has distinctive "punched-out" areas of bone destruction, which are usually consistent in size, whereas the ribs may have lacelike areas of bone destruction and small osteolytic lesions, which are sometimes associated by nearby soft tissue masses. The flat and long bones have areas of medullary bone destruction, and if they arise around the cortex, they are followed by scalloping of the inner cortical margin (Figs. 8.5 and 8.6).

Fig. 8.5 Radiograph of skull showing typical punched out lesions without sclerosis with uniform size

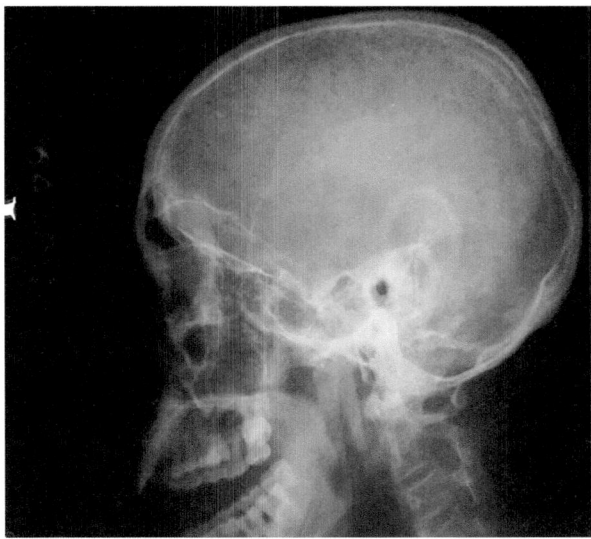

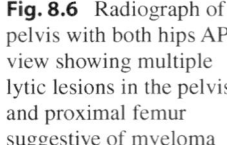

Fig. 8.6 Radiograph of pelvis with both hips AP view showing multiple lytic lesions in the pelvis and proximal femur suggestive of myeloma

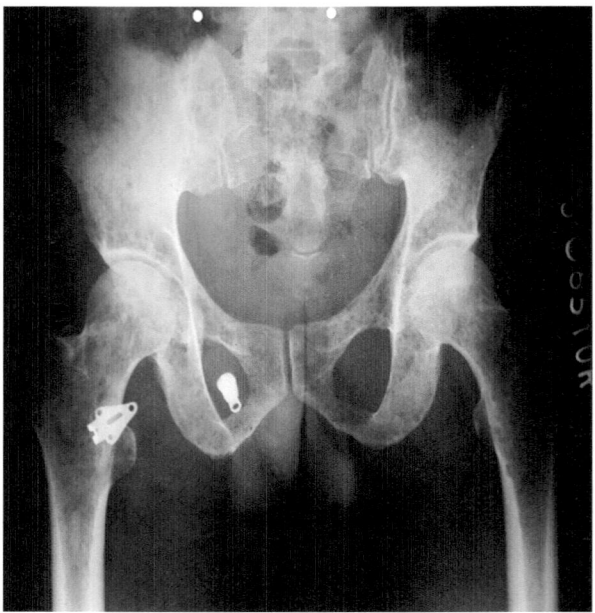

8.5   Adamantinoma

Adamantinoma is an uncommon malignant tumour that affects both men and women in their second and fifth decades of life, with 90% of cases involving the tibia. The tumour is distinguished radiographically by well-defined and elongated osteolytic lesions of varied sizes, separated by patches of sclerotic bone that occasionally give the lesion a "soap bubble" look; there is usually no periosteal reaction (Fig. 8.7).

Fig. 8.7 Lateral radiograph of tibia showing a lytic lesion in the mid-diaphysis of tibia with reactive sclerosis with soap bubble appearance suggestive of adamantinoma

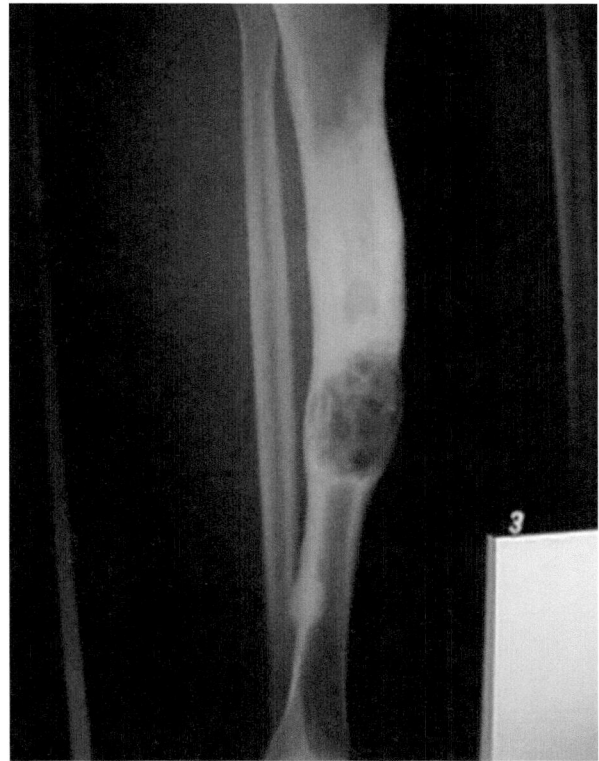

Bibliography

1. Greenspan A Beltran J. *Orthopedic Imaging : A Practical Approach*. Sixth ed. Philadelphia: Wolters Kluwer; 2015.
2. Picci P, Manfrini M, Fabbri N, et al., editors. Atlas of musculoskeletal tumors and tumorlike lesions: the Rizzolo case archive. Cham: Springer; 2020.
3. Yochum TR Rowe LJ. *Yochum and Rowe's Essentials of Skeletal Radiology*. 3rd ed. Philadelphia: Lippincott/Williams & Wilkins; 2005.

Radiographs of Metastatic Bone Tumours

Compared to primary bone tumours, skeletal metastases from carcinomas happen far more frequently. In most cases, malignant cells grow inside the bone, replace the healthy bone marrow, and destroy the bone. Metastases from prostate and some breast cancers promote the growth of neoplastic bone. Although almost all malignant tumours have the capacity to spread to the bone, carcinomas of the breast, lung, prostate, kidney, and thyroid are the most frequently occurring. Prostate, lung, or breast cancer patients are more likely than the general population to get bone metastases. In patients with metastatic bone disease, the tumour must erode between 30 and 50% of the bone for the lesion to be seen on a plain radiograph. A technetium bone scan is a more accurate way to find metastatic illness, but it may not be accurate for tumours that spread quickly, including multiple myeloma or renal cell carcinoma. The majority of metastases break down bone; however those from prostate and breast tumours can promote bone growth and show up on plain radiographs as areas of increased bone density (Figs. 9.1 and 9.2).

© The Author(s), under exclusive license to Springer Nature Singapore Pte Ltd. 2023
N. S. Kushwaha, M. B. Abbas, *A Guide to Musculoskeletal Radiology*,
https://doi.org/10.1007/978-981-99-6155-9_9

Fig. 9.1 AP view of the pelvis showing multiple lytic lesions in the pelvis and proximal femur. (Metastasis)

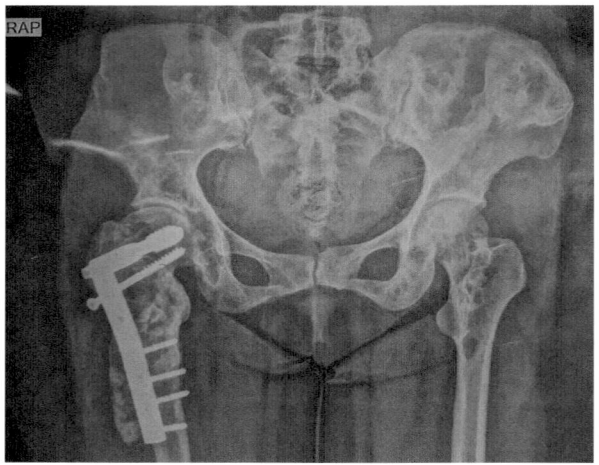

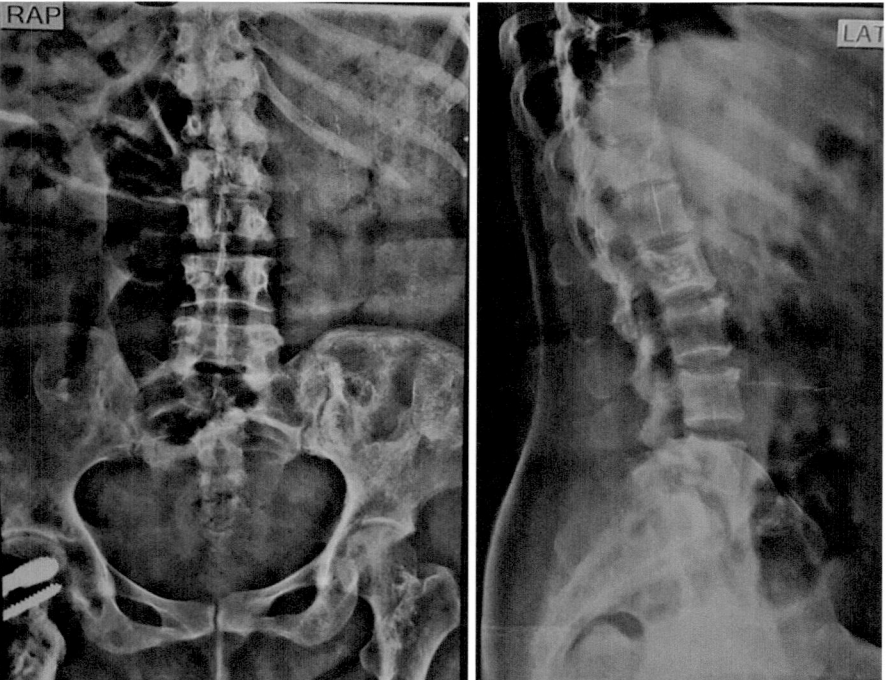

Fig. 9.2 AP and lateral view of lumbar spine showing lytic lesions on T12 and L2 vertebrae suggestive of metastasis

Bibliography

1. Greenspan A Beltran J. *Orthopedic Imaging: A Practical Approach.* Sixth ed. Philadelphia: Wolters Kluwer; 2015.
2. Picci P, Manfrini M, Fabbri N, et al., editors. Atlas of musculoskeletal tumors and tumorlike lesions: the Rizzolo case archive. Cham: Springer; 2020.
3. Yochum TR, Rowe LJ. *Yochum and Rowe's Essentials of Skeletal Radiology.* 3rd ed. Philadelphia: Lippincott/Williams & Wilkins; 2005.

Radiographs of Upper Extremity Diseases

10

10.1 Osteoarthritis of Shoulder

Primary arthritis of shoulder joint is rare. One must rule out secondary causes of arthritis before diagnosing it as a case of idiopathic arthritis (Fig. 10.1).

© The Author(s), under exclusive license to Springer Nature Singapore Pte Ltd. 2023
N. S. Kushwaha, M. B. Abbas, *A Guide to Musculoskeletal Radiology*,
https://doi.org/10.1007/978-981-99-6155-9_10

Fig. 10.1 Anteroposterior radiograph of shoulder showing osteoarthritis of shoulder joint with reduced joint space, subchondral sclerosis, and irregular joint line

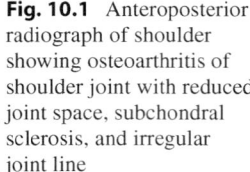

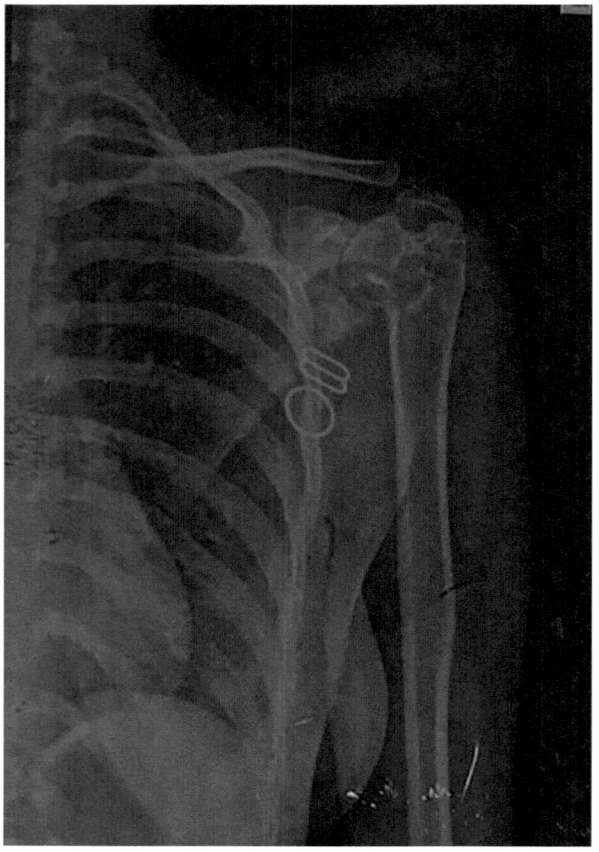

Bibliography

1. Greenspan A Beltran J. *Orthopedic Imaging: A Practical Approach.* Sixth ed. Philadelphia: Wolters Kluwer; 2015.
2. Eisenberg RL. Clinical imaging: an atlas of clinical diagnosis. 5th ed. Philadelphia: Wolters Kluwer/Lippincott Williams & Wilkins; 2010.

Radiographs of Lower Extremity Diseases

11

11.1 Osteoarthritis

The most prevalent type of arthritis is degenerative joint disease, often known as osteoarthritis or osteoarthrosis. Osteoarthritis typically affects people over the age of 50 in its original (idiopathic) form; but, in its secondary form, it can afflict people much younger than this. Patients in the latter group have well-defined underlying diseases that cause degenerative joint disease to develop.

11.2 Osteoarthritis of Hip

Four key radiographic signs of degenerative joint disease in the hip are as follows:

- Articular cartilage thinning, which results in a narrowing of the joint space.
- Subchondral sclerosis (eburnation) brought on by healing (remodelling) processes.
- Osteophyte development (osteophytosis) results from reparative processes in low-stress zones, which are often marginal (peripheral) in distribution and not susceptible to stress.
- Eggers cysts are subchondral cyst-like lesions that develop in the acetabulum and are caused by bone contusions that cause microfractures and the infiltration of synovial fluid into the changed spongy bone (Fig. 11.1).

Patients with predisposing conditions, such as prior trauma, femoroacetabular impingement (FAI) syndrome, slipped capital femoral epiphysis, congenital hip dislocation, Perthes disease, osteonecrosis, Paget disease, and inflammatory arthritides, frequently develop secondary osteoarthritis in the hip joint. The characteristics

© The Author(s), under exclusive license to Springer Nature Singapore Pte Ltd. 2023
N. S. Kushwaha, M. B. Abbas, *A Guide to Musculoskeletal Radiology*,
https://doi.org/10.1007/978-981-99-6155-9_11

Fig. 11.1 Anteroposterior radiograph of the hip demonstrates the radiographic hallmarks of osteoarthritis: narrowing of the joint space, particularly at the weight-bearing area, formation of marginal osteophytes, and subchondral sclerosis

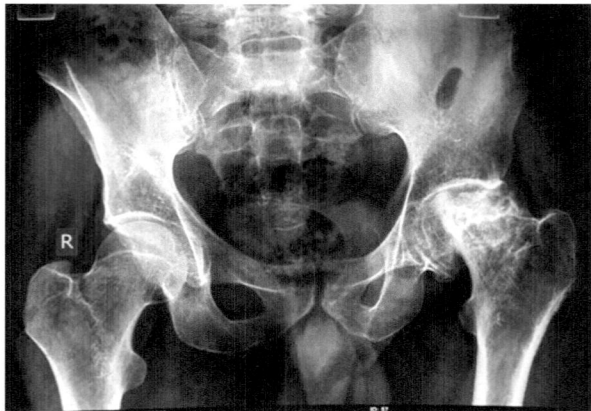

of the underlying process can frequently be seen in addition to the radiographic results, which are the same as those described for primary osteoarthritis. Although the typical radiographic views are usually sufficient for demonstrating these changes, a more precise evaluation of the condition of the articular cartilage may occasionally need a CT scan, arthrography, or an MRI.

11.3   Osteoarthritis of Knee

The medial femorotibial, lateral femorotibial, and femoropatellar compartments, which make up the knee's three main compartments, are each susceptible to degenerative changes. These alterations have similar radiographic characteristics to osteoarthritis of the hip, such as narrowing of the joint space (typically one or two compartments), subchondral sclerosis, osteophytosis, and the development of subchondral cysts (or pseudocysts). These processes can be shown by using the knee's typical lateral and anteroposterior projections. Involvement of the lateral compartment may result in a valgus configuration, which is best illustrated on the weight-bearing anteroposterior view. If the medial joint compartment is damaged, the knee may acquire a varus configuration (Fig. 11.2).

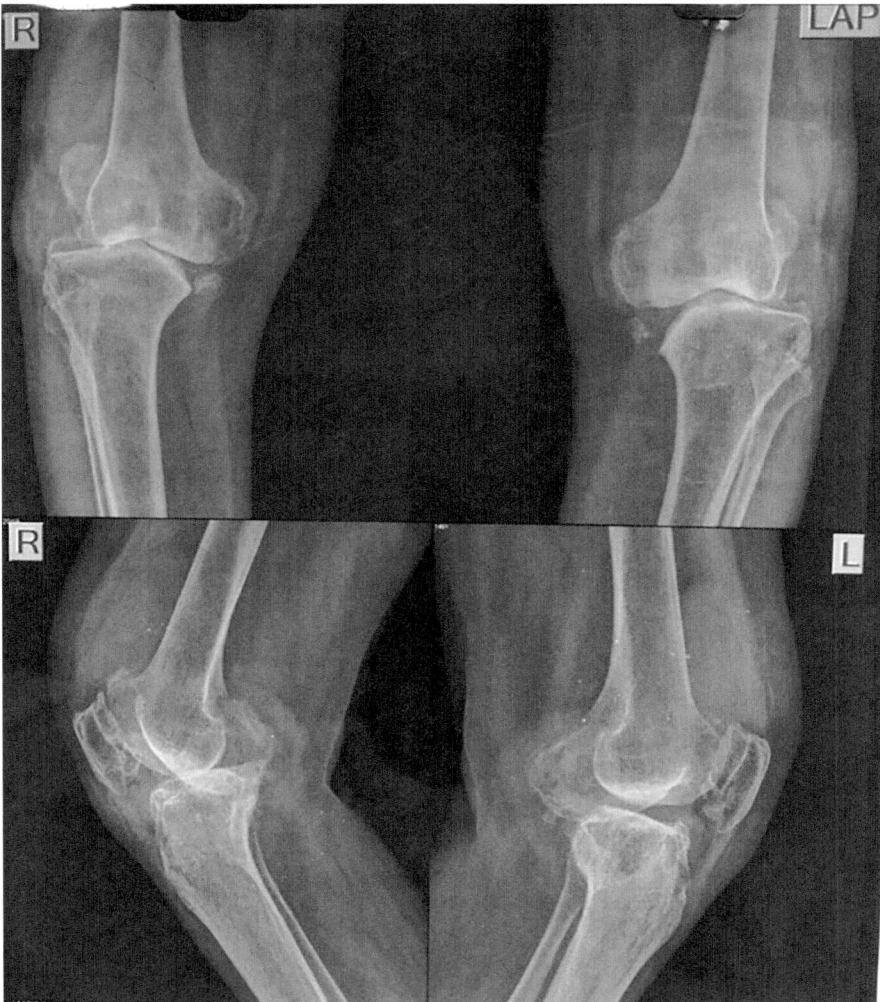

Fig. 11.2 AP and lateral radiographs of bilateral knee demonstrating narrowing of the medial femorotibial and femoropatellar compartments, subchondral sclerosis, and osteophytosis, which are the typical features of osteoarthritis

11.4   Osteoarthritis of Ankle

Osteoarthritis, post-traumatic arthritis, and inflammatory arthritis are the three main kinds of ankle arthritis, which affects the tibiotalar joint. Plain radiographs of the ankle are the main diagnostic tool. Loss of joint space, subchondral sclerosis and cysts, eburnation, and potential angular deformity are all radiographic findings (Fig. 11.3).

Fig. 11.3 AP and lateral
view of ankle joint
showing decreased joint
space with subchondral
sclerosis typical of ankle
joint arthritis

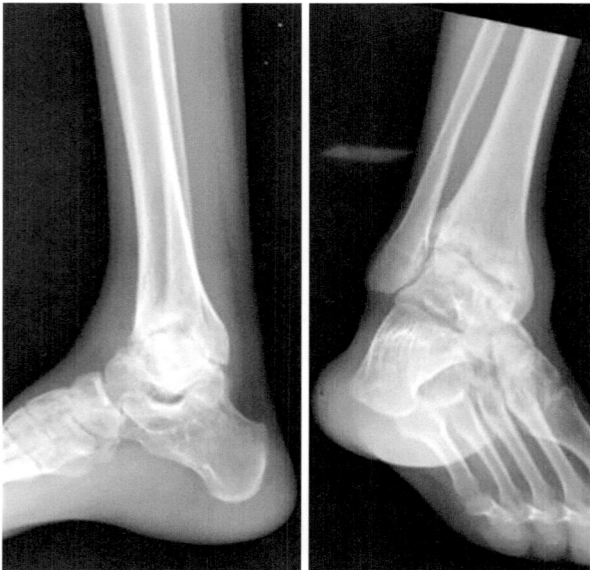

Bibliography

1. Greenspan A Beltran J. *Orthopedic Imaging: A Practical Approach*. Sixth ed. Philadelphia: Wolters Kluwer; 2015.
2. Eisenberg RL. Clinical imaging: an atlas of clinical diagnosis. 5th ed. Philadelphia: Wolters Kluwer/Lippincott Williams & Wilkins; 2010.

Radiographs of Spine Region (Deformity)

12.1 Scoliosis

A lateral curvature of the spine that occurs in the coronal plane is referred to as scoliosis. This sets it apart from lordosis, which is an anterior curvature of the spine in the sagittal plane, and kyphosis, which is a posterior curvature of the spine in the sagittal plane. The curvature is referred to as kyphoscoliosis if it is present in both the coronal and sagittal planes. Scoliosis can also have a rotational component, in which the vertebrae rotate in the direction of the convexity of the curve.

Three classifications can be used to categorise idiopathic scoliosis, which makes up over 70% of all scoliotic anomalies. The infantile form, of which there are two varieties, affects children under the age of four. It is more common in boys, and the thoracic segment typically exhibits a left-sided convexity. In the resolving (benign) variety, the curve typically doesn't rise over 30° and resolves on its own without the need for intervention. Without vigorous therapy starting early in the process, the progressive variety has a poor prognosis and the potential for severe deformity. Between the ages of 4 and 9 years old, both boys and girls can develop juvenile idiopathic scoliosis. The teenage form of idiopathic scoliosis, which accounts for 85% of occurrences and is primarily found in girls between the ages of 10 and skeletal maturity, is by far the most prevalent kind. Most frequently, the thoracic or thoracolumbar spine is affected, and the curve is convex to the right.

Approximately 10% of cases of this deformity are due to congenital scoliosis. Generally speaking, it can be divided into three groups, according to MacEwen: those resulting from a failure in vertebral formation, which can be partial or complete; those caused by a failure in vertebral segmentation, which can be asymmetric and unilateral or symmetric and bilateral; and those resulting from a combination of the first two.

Radiographic examination involves standing anteroposterior and lateral radiographs of the complete spine, a supine anteroposterior film focused over the

N. S. Kushwaha, M. B. Abbas, *A Guide to Musculoskeletal Radiology*, https://doi.org/10.1007/978-981-99-6155-9_12

103

scoliotic curve, which is utilised for the various measurements of spinal curvature and vertebral rotation, and anteroposterior radiographs taken with the patient bending laterally to either side for evaluation of the flexible and structural components of the curve. For the purpose of determining skeletal maturity, care should be taken to ensure that the iliac crests are visible in at least one of these radiographs (Figs. 12.1, 12.2 and 12.3).

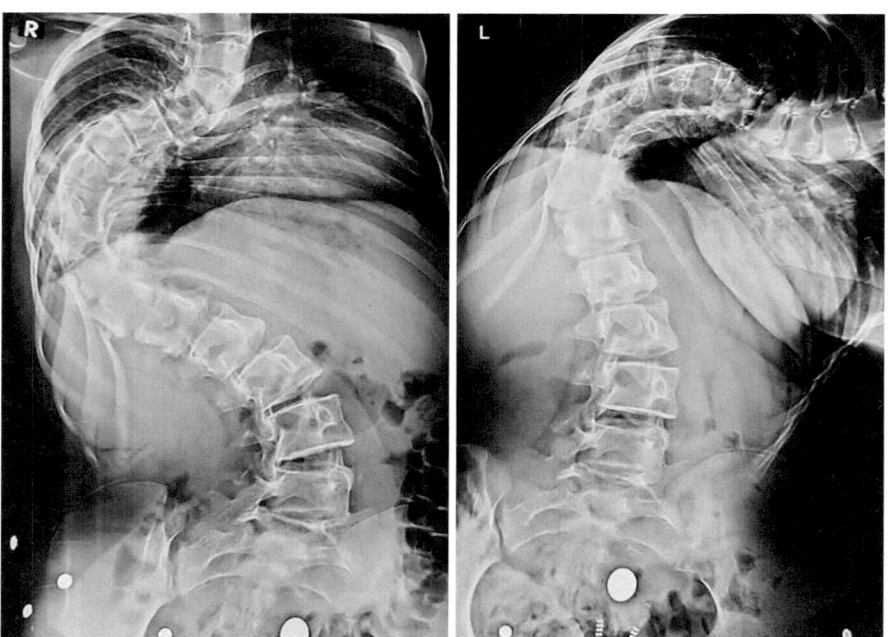

Fig. 12.1 Anteroposterior radiograph of the spine shows the typical features of idiopathic scoliosis involving the thoracolumbar segment. The convexity of the curve is to the right; a compensatory curve in the lumbar segment has its convexity to the left

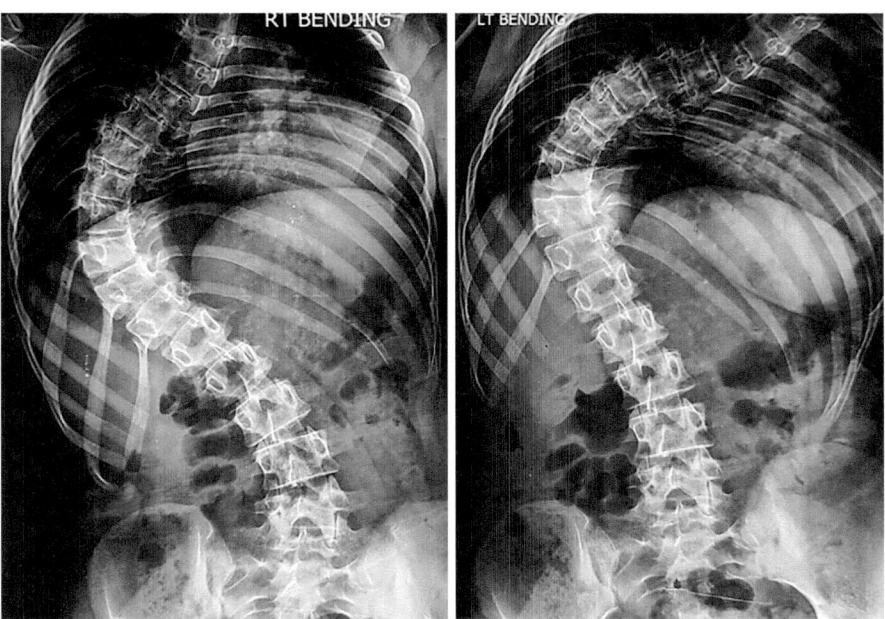

Fig. 12.2   Anteroposterior radiograph of thoracolumbar spine showing idiopathic scoliosis of thoracolumbar spine with convexity towards the right side

Fig. 12.3 Calculation of Cobb's angle (angle of scoliosis): The vertebrae towards the end of the structural curve are those that tilt into the concavity of the curve the most. The vertebra whose centre is most lateral from the central line is the apical one, which exhibits the most severe rotation and wedging. A tangent line is drawn from the upper surface of the upper end vertebra and lower surface of the lower end vertebra. A perpendicular line is drawn from both of these lines and the intersection forms an angle known as scoliotic angle

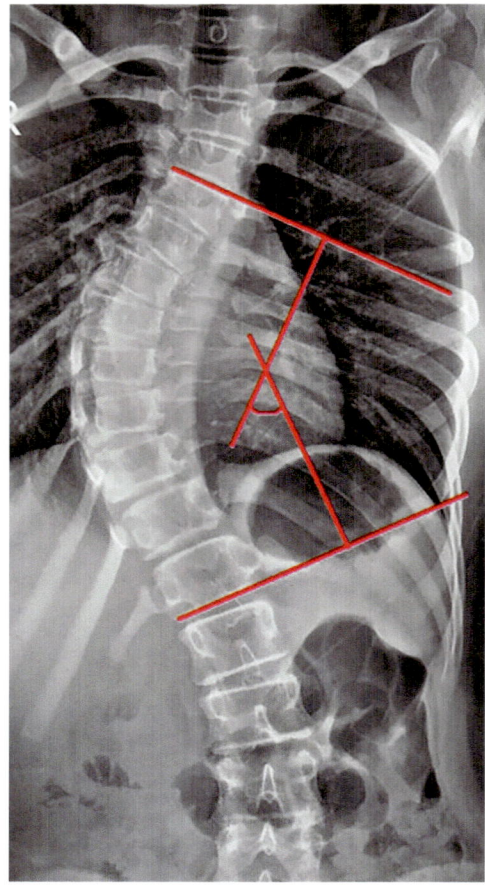

Bibliography

1. Greenspan A Beltran J. *Orthopedic Imaging: A Practical Approach.* Sixth ed. Philadelphia: Wolters Kluwer; 2015.
2. Eisenberg RL. Clinical imaging: an atlas of clinical diagnosis. 5th ed. Philadelphia: Wolters Kluwer/Lippincott Williams & Wilkins; 2010.

Radiographs of Congenital and Developmental Skeletal Disorders

13

Formation anomalies can also be found in bone, such as pseudoarthroses and bone fusions (syndactyly and synostosis). Abnormalities in the size or shape of bones can result from disruptions in bone growth. Undergrowth (hypoplasia or atrophy), overgrowth (hypertrophy or gigantism), or distorted growth, such as congenital tibia vara, are all possible outcomes. Contractures, subluxations, and dislocations are all examples of anomalies affecting joint motion caused by bone development abnormalities. Those with abnormalities in bone growth, maturation, and modelling, as manifested in the various dysplasias, are among the last group of congenital defects affecting the skeletal system.

The diagnosis can usually be made using standard radiographic projections relevant to the anatomic site under examination. Radiographs should be taken in at least two projections at 90° to one another, as with most other orthopaedic conditions. Supplemental views, on the other hand, are sometimes required for a complete examination of an anomaly, especially when it involves complex structures like the ankle and foot. When possible, weight-bearing radiographs of the foot should be taken (Figs. 13.1, 13.2, 13.3, 13.4, 13.5, 13.6, 13.7, 13.8, 13.9, 13.10, 13.11, 13.12, 13.13 and 13.14).

© The Author(s), under exclusive license to Springer Nature Singapore Pte Ltd. 2023
N. S. Kushwaha, M. B. Abbas, *A Guide to Musculoskeletal Radiology*,
https://doi.org/10.1007/978-981-99-6155-9_13

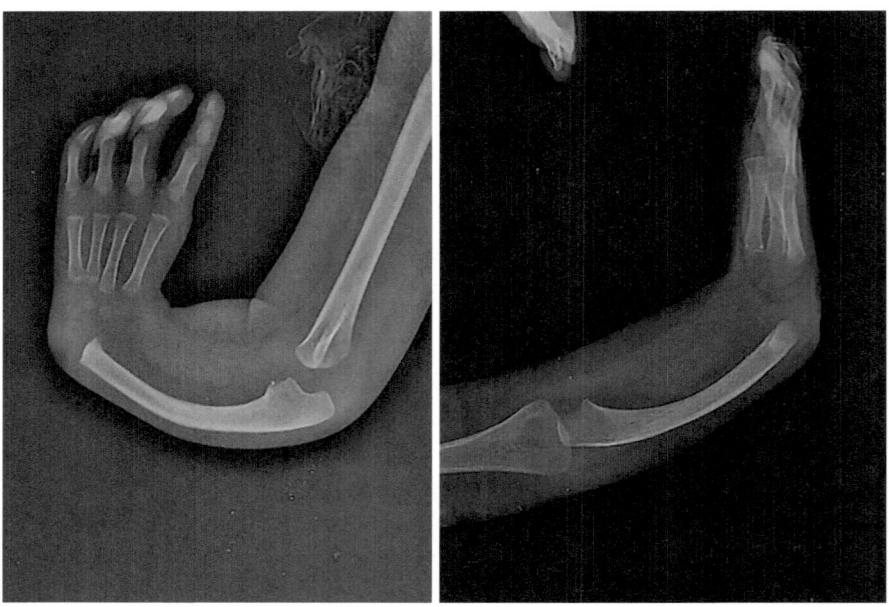

Fig. 13.1   AP and lateral view of forearm showing absence of radius (radial amelia)

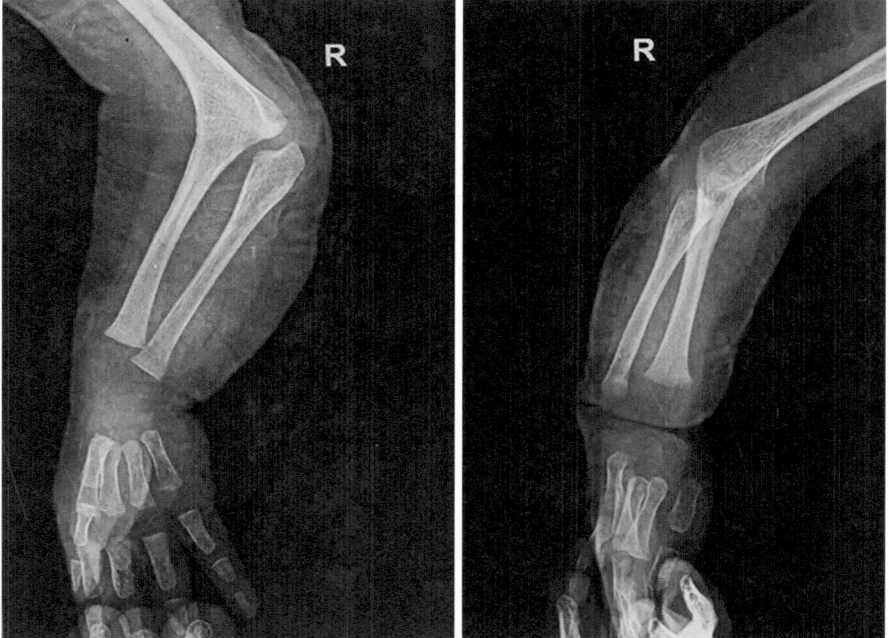

Fig. 13.2   AP and lateral view if elbow showing humeroradial synostosis

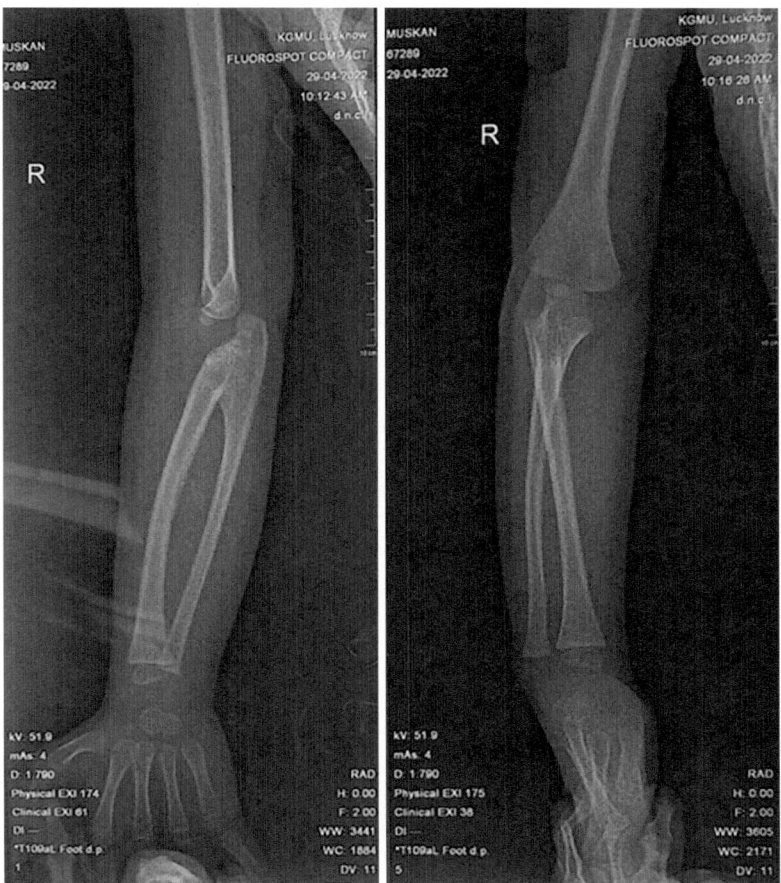

Fig. 13.3 AP and lateral view of forearm showing radioulnar synostosis

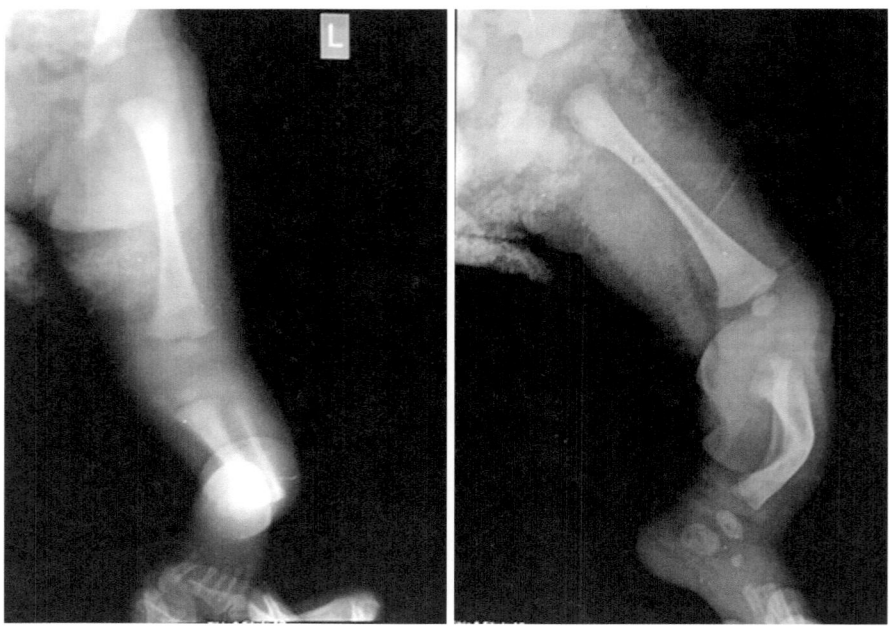

Fig. 13.4 AP lateral view of leg showing congenital anterolateral bowing of tibia

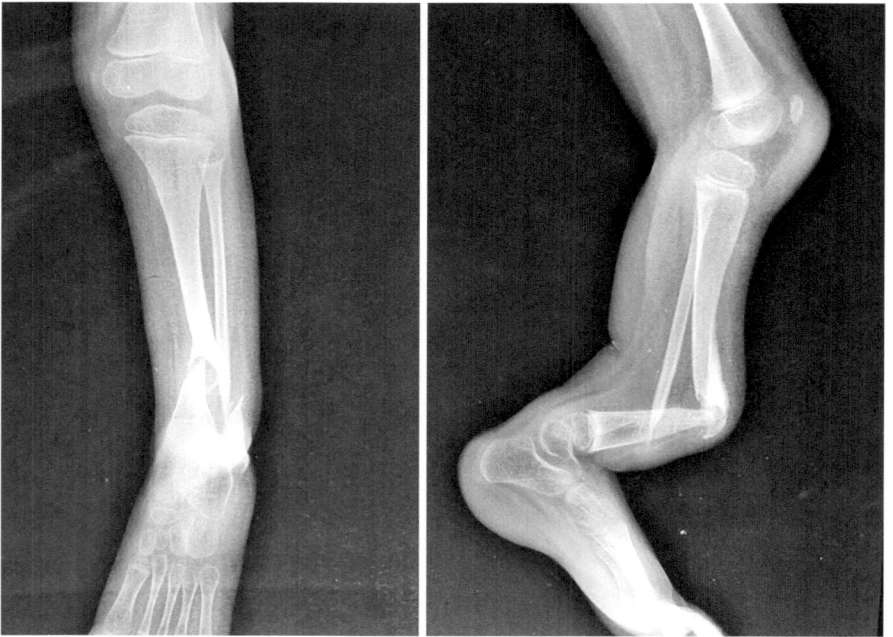

Fig. 13.5 AP and lateral view of leg showing congenital pseudoarthrosis of tibia

Fig. 13.6 AP view of pelvis showing bilateral congenital dislocation of hip

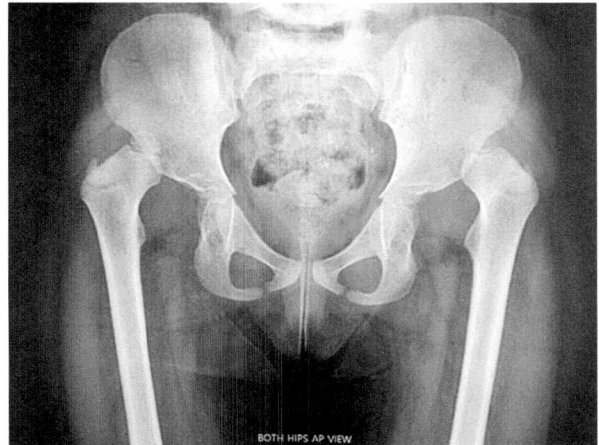

Fig. 13.7 AP view of pelvis showing developmental dysplasia of right hip joint

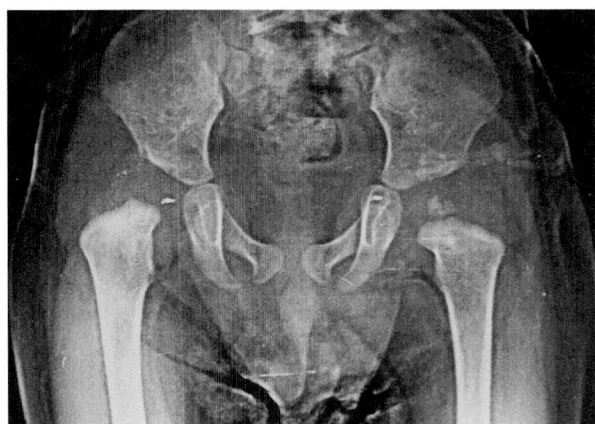

Fig. 13.8 AP view of pelvis showing congenital coxa vara of left hip

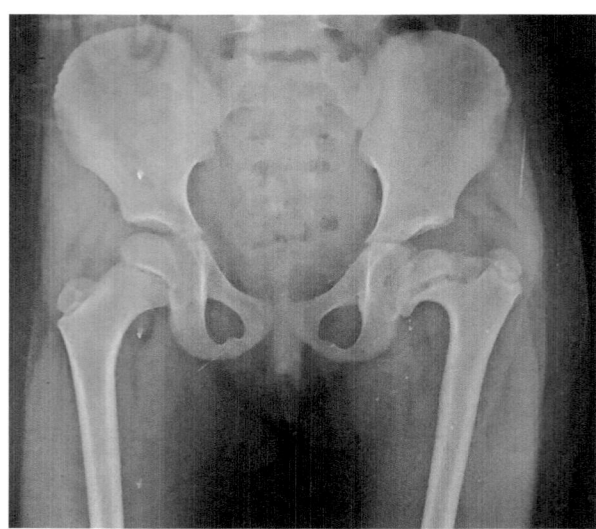

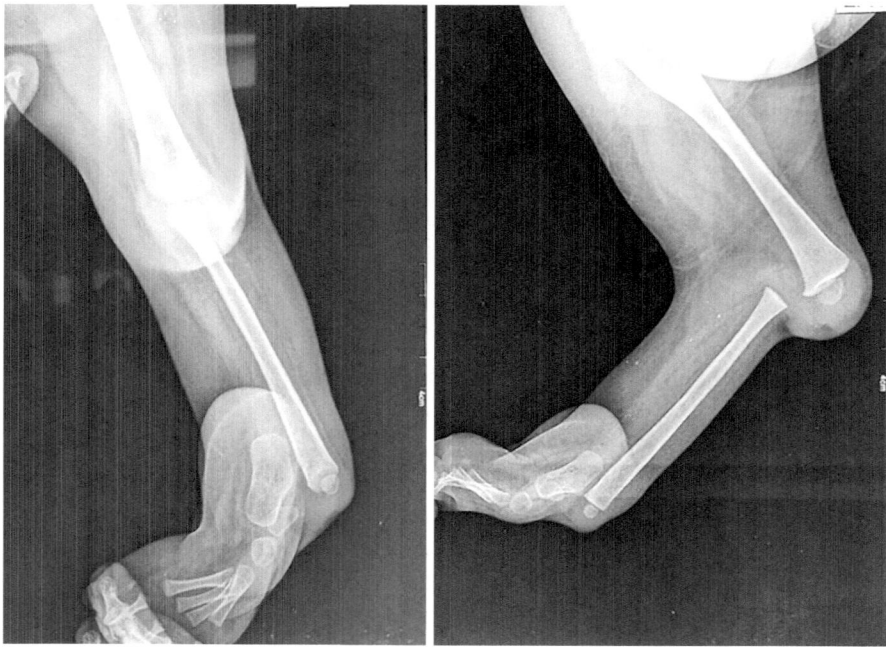

Fig. 13.9 AP and lateral view of leg showing tibial amelia

Fig. 13.10 AP and lateral view of right lower limb showing absence of femur bone (proximal femur focal deficiency)

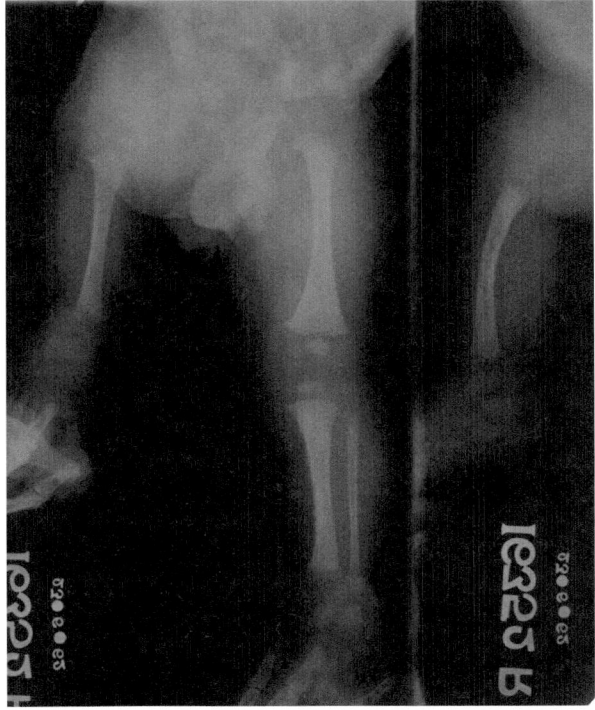

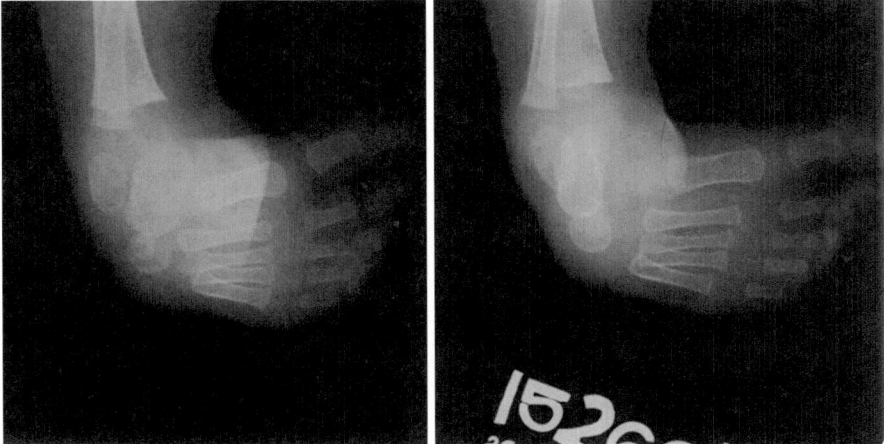

Fig. 13.11 X-ray of foot showing congenital talipes equinovarus

Fig. 13.12 AP view of pelvis showing bilateral congenital coxa vara

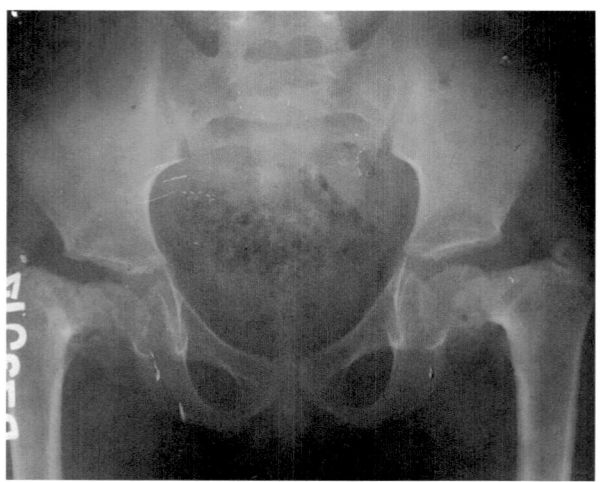

Fig. 13.13 AP view of dorso-lumbar spine showing scoliosis (adolescent idiopathic scoliosis)

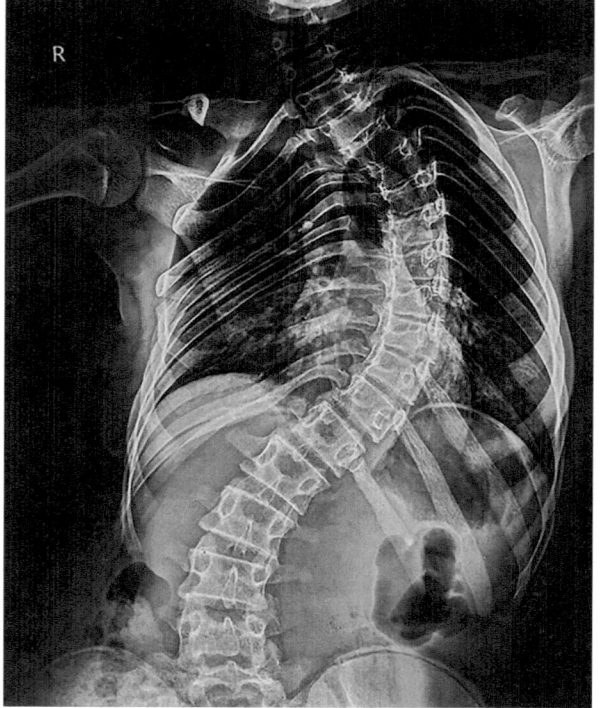

Fig. 13.14 AP view of
wrist showing volar medial
physeal damage with
growth arrest (madelung
deformity)

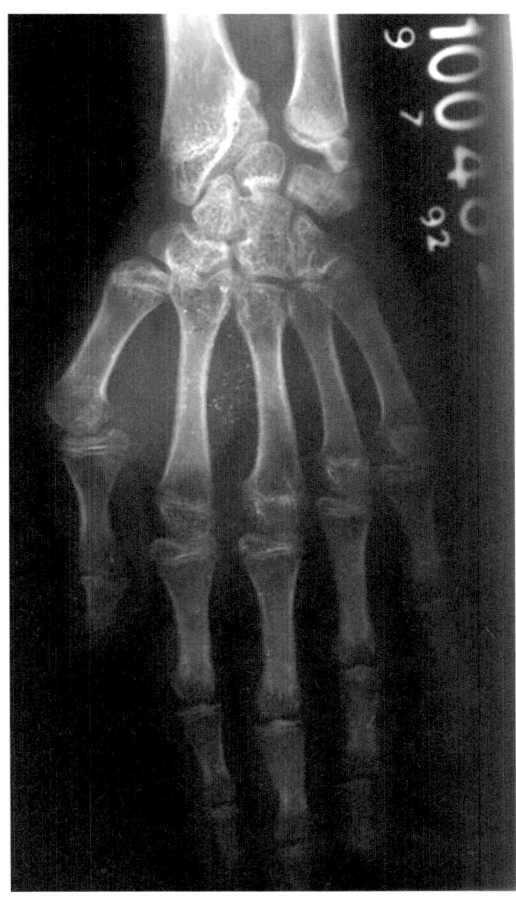

Bibliography

1. Yochum TR, Rowe LJ. *Yochum and Rowe's Essentials of Skeletal Radiology*. 3rd ed.
   Philadelphia: Lippincott/Williams & Wilkins; 2005.

Part V

Musculoskeletal Infections

Radiographs of Musculoskeletal Infections

14

Infections of the musculoskeletal system can be divided into three types: bone infections (osteomyelitis), joint infections (infectious arthritis), and soft tissue infections (cellulitis).

14.1 Pyogenic Osteomyelitis

Soft tissue oedema and loss of fascial planes are the first radiological indicators of bone infection. These normally appear within 24 to 48 h of the commencement of the infection. Evidence of a destructive lytic lesion is present usually within 7 to 10 days following the onset of infection, and a positive radionuclide bone scan are the first changes in the bone. Progressive breakdown of cortical and medullary bone, increased endosteal sclerosis indicating reactive new bone formation, and a periosteal reaction occur between 2 and 6 weeks. Sequestra, which indicate patches of necrotic bone, normally appear in 6 to 8 weeks and are surrounded by a dense involucrum, which represents a sheath of periosteal new bone (Figs. 14.1, 14.2, 14.3 and 14.4).

© The Author(s), under exclusive license to Springer Nature Singapore Pte Ltd. 2023
N. S. Kushwaha, M. B. Abbas, *A Guide to Musculoskeletal Radiology*,
https://doi.org/10.1007/978-981-99-6155-9_14

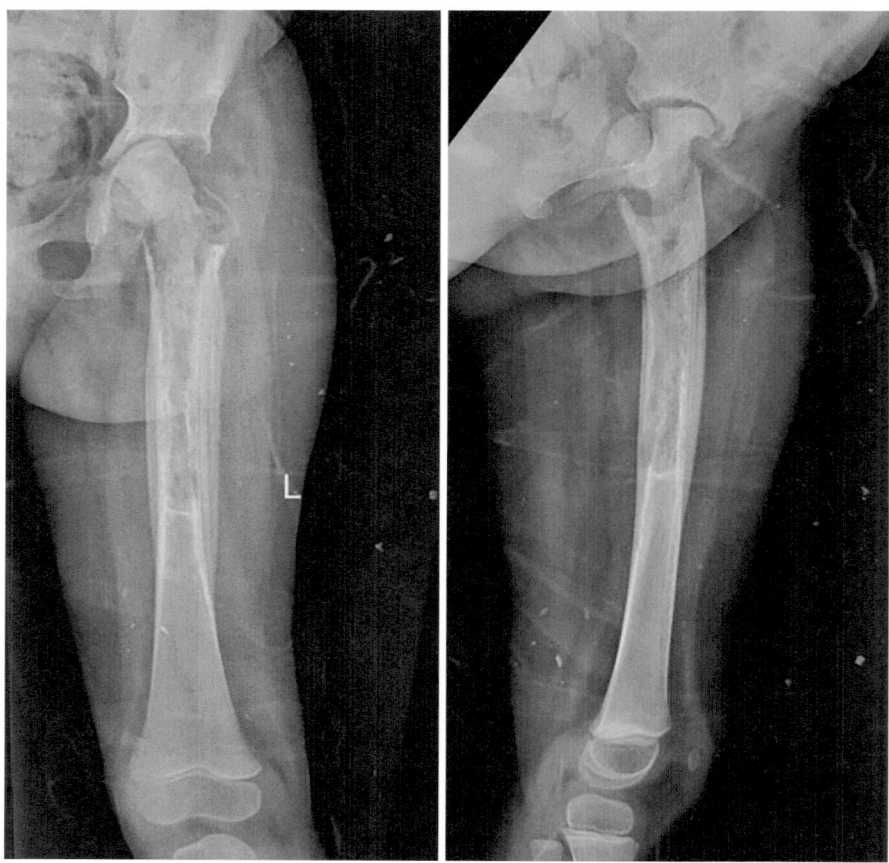

Fig. 14.1 X-ray shows cortical and medullary bone destruction of proximal half of femur with periosteal reaction, involucrum, and sequestrum formation suggestive of chronic osteomyelitis

Fig. 14.2 X-ray of femur
showing medullary bone
destruction in the
mid-diaphysis with
periosteal reaction with
sequestrum formation
suggestive of chronic
osteomyelitis

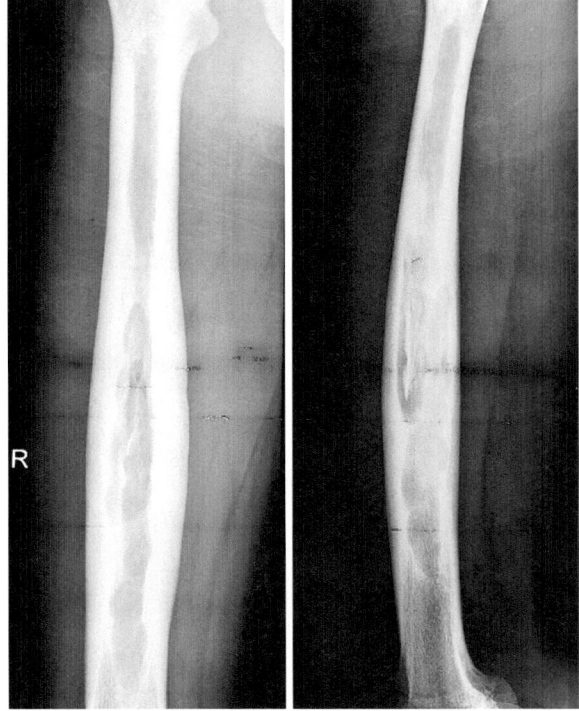

Fig. 14.3 X-ray of
forearm showing cortical
and medullary bone
destruction of mid-
diaphysis of ulna with
periosteal reaction and
sequestrum formation

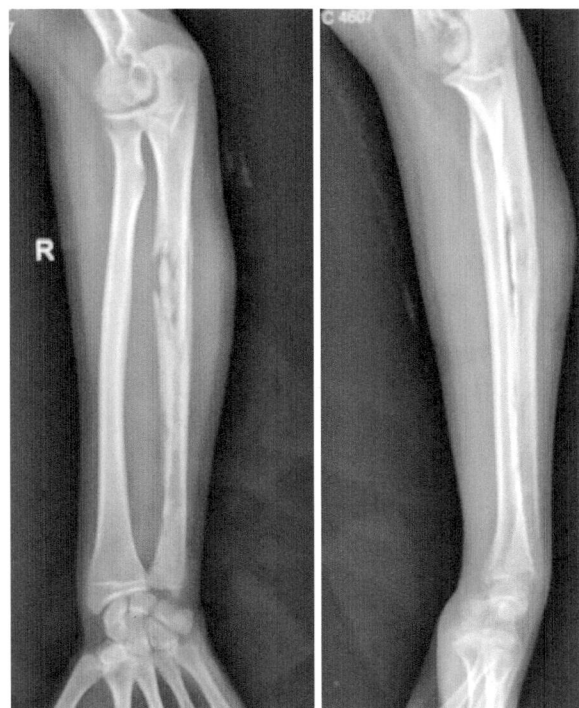

Fig. 14.4 X-ray of leg
showing cortical and
medullary destruction of
tibia with periosteal
reaction and sequestrum
formation

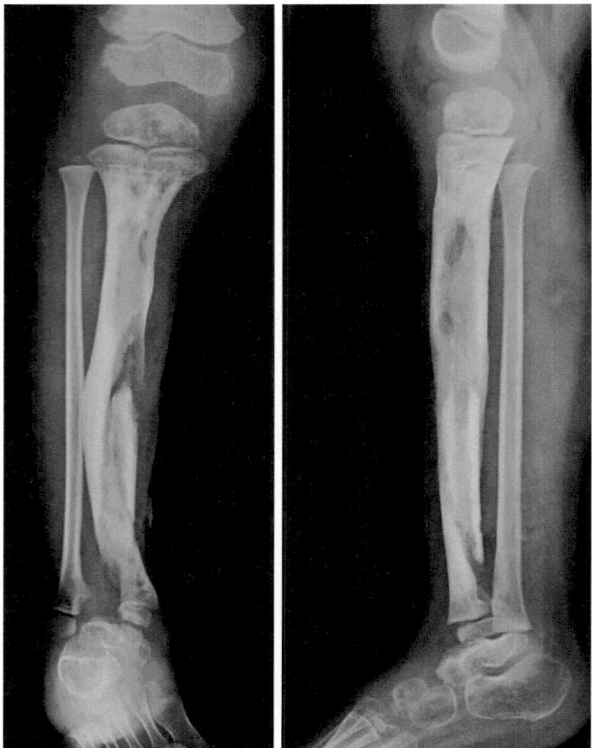

14.2   Infectious Arthritis

Septic arthritis is commonly diagnosed with conventional radiography. Certain radiographic findings may aid in making the accurate diagnosis. A single joint, usually a weight-bearing joint like the knee or hip, is usually affected. Joint effusion, soft tissue swelling, and periarticular osteoporosis are common early signs of joint infection, but on X-ray joint space is frequently preserved. Articular cartilage is damaged in the later stages of pyogenic arthritis; both subarticular plates are typically involved, and the joint space narrows.

The Phemister triad, which includes periarticular osteoporosis, peripheral osseous erosions, and gradual narrowing of the joint space, is characteristic of tuberculosis of a peripheral joint, which usually manifests as a monoarticular disease (Fig. 14.5).

Fig. 14.5 X-ray pelvis with both hip showing joint space narrowing of left hip joint with juxta-articular osteopenia with subchondral bony destruction suggestive of septic arthritis

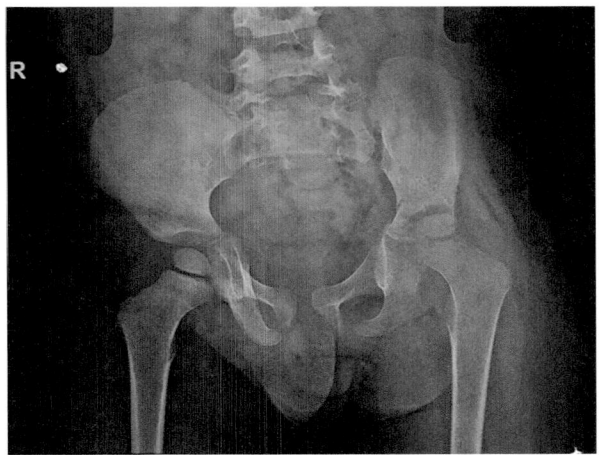

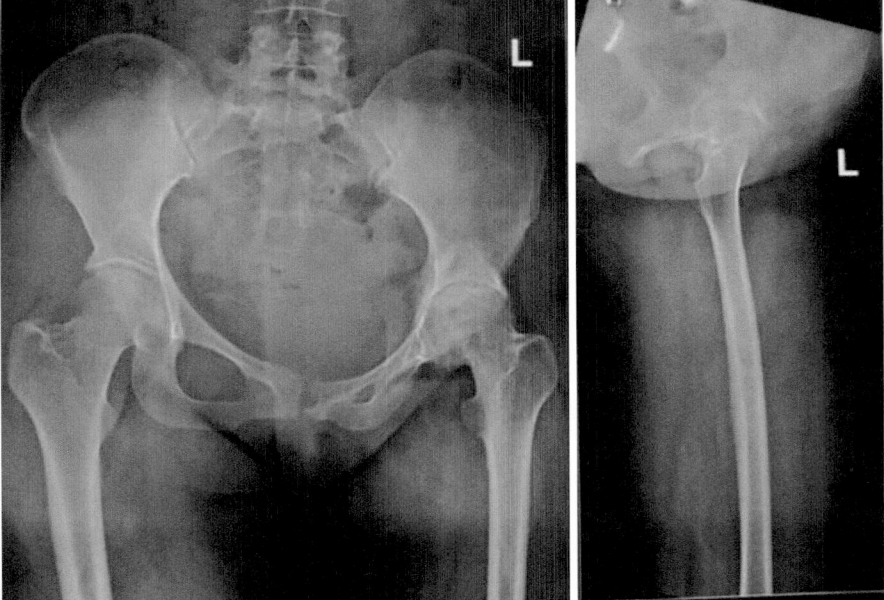

X-ray pelvis with both hip showing reduced joint space with juxta-articular osteoporosis and bony erosions in head of femur and acetabulum suggestive of tubercular infectious arthritis (Figs. 14.6 and 14.7).

Fig. 14.6 X-ray pelvis with both hip showing reduced joint space with sclerosis of head of femur and acetabular roof suggestive of tubercular arthritis of left hip joint (post-ATT)

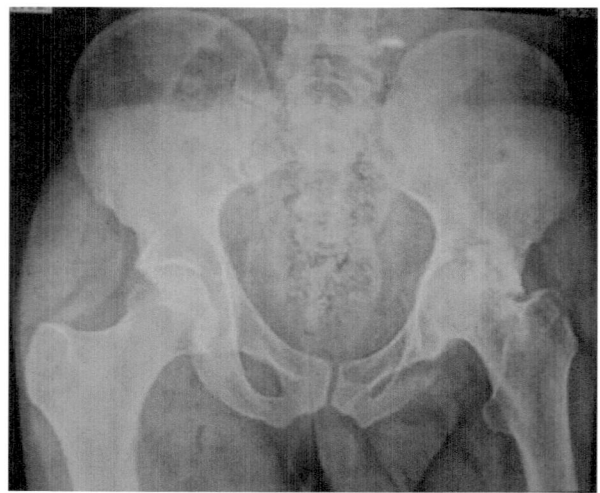

Fig. 14.7 X-ray pelvis with both hip showing mortar pestle appearance of right hip joint suggestive of tuberculosis

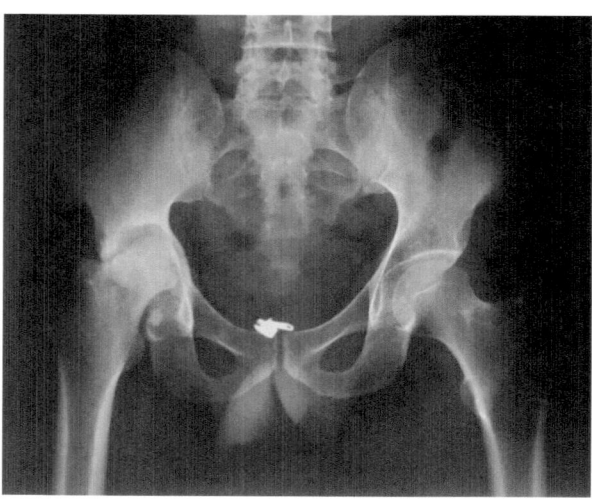

14.3   Tuberculosis of Spine

Tuberculous spondylitis, also known as Pott's spine, is an infection of the spine caused by the tubercle bacillus. The vertebral body or intervertebral disc may be infected, with infection most commonly occurring in the lower thoracic and upper lumbar vertebrae. The disease accounts for 25% to 50% of all skeletal TB cases. The imaging characteristics of tuberculous infection of the spine resemble those of pyogenic infections. The disc space is narrowing, and the end plates of the vertebrae next to the affected disc show signs of damage. A paraspinal mass is a common occurrence. The infectious process can occasionally damage a single vertebra or a portion of a vertebra (pedicle) without invading the disc (Figs. 14.8 and 14.9).

Fig. 14.8 Anteroposterior and lateral radiograph of spine showing reduced joint space between D10 and D11 vertebrae with end plate erosion and paraspinal soft tissue shadow (bird's nest abscess) suggestive of Pott's spine

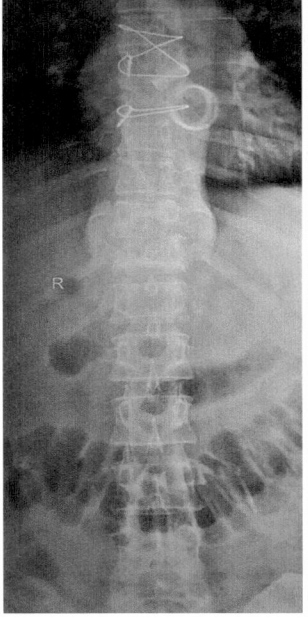
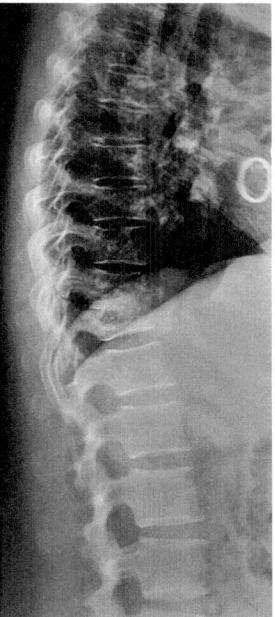

Fig. 14.9 Anteroposterior and lateral radiograph of spine showing reduced joint space between D10 and D11 vertebrae with end plate erosion and paraspinal soft tissue shadow (bird's nest abscess) suggestive of Pott's spine

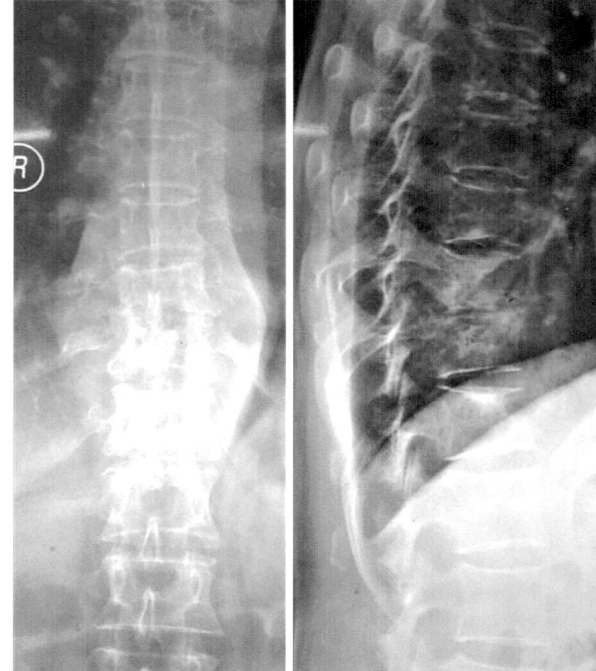

Bibliography

1. Yochum TR, Rowe LJ. *Yochum and Rowe's Essentials of Skeletal Radiology*. 3rd ed. Philadelphia: Lippincott/Williams & Wilkins; 2005.
2. Greenspan A Beltran J. *Orthopedic Imaging: A Practical Approach*. Sixth ed. Philadelphia: Wolters Kluwer; 2015.

Part VI

Metabolic and Endocrine Skeletal Disorders

Radiographs of Metabolic and Endocrine Skeletal Disorders

15

Radiographically, anomalies in bone density that are typically associated with increased bone formation, increased bone resorption, or insufficient bone mineralisation describe the majority of metabolic and endocrine disorders. Osteopenia or radiodensity are two aberrant radiographic features of the afflicted bones (osteosclerosis).

The simplest and most popular technique for determining bone density is radiography. This method is capable of picking up even the smallest increases in bone density, but it typically misses losses in overall skeletal mineralisation until they are at least 30% lower. It must be noted that due to technical mistakes, such as incorrect milliamperage and kilovoltage settings, normal bone might quickly take on an aberrant radiographic appearance. For instance, increased bone radiolucency appears to be caused by overexposure, whereas artificially increased bone radiodensity results from underexposure.

Because this result is not specific to osteoporosis, osteomalacia, or hyperparathyroidism, it should not be referred to as osteoporosis when it appears relative to increased bone radiolucency on routine radiographs. Most experts concur that osteopenia is the term that best describes increasing radiolucency (poverty of bone). Both disorders are characterised by increased bone radiolucency, with osteoporosis specifically referring to a reduction in the amount of bone tissue (deficient bone matrix) and osteomalacia specifically referring to a reduction in the amount of mineral in the matrix (deficient mineralisation).

© The Author(s), under exclusive license to Springer Nature Singapore Pte Ltd. 2023
N. S. Kushwaha, M. B. Abbas, *A Guide to Musculoskeletal Radiology*,
https://doi.org/10.1007/978-981-99-6155-9_15

15.1   Osteoporosis

Osteoporosis is a metabolic bone disease that affects the entire body, causing decreased bone mass and microstructural degradation of bone. It is defined by insufficient production or excessive resorption of bone matrix. Even though there is less bone tissue overall, what is still there is totally calcified. To put it another way, the bone has a numeric deficiency but a qualitative one.

15.2   Rickets and Osteomalacia

While decreasing bone mass is the primary change in osteoporosis, defective mineralisation (calcification) of the bone matrix is the primary bone abnormality in rickets, which affects children, and osteomalacia, which affects adults. Osteoid tissue cannot properly calcify if sufficient supplies of calcium and phosphorus are not present.

Infantile rickets is characterised by extensive skeletal demineralisation, which causes weight-bearing bones to bend when newborns start to stand and walk. Early-stage rickets infants have trouble sleeping and are agitated. The fontanelles' closure is postponed. The cranial vault begins to soften as the first physical symptom (craniotabes). The costochondral junction's cartilage enlargement results in the rachitic rosary prominence. Alkaline phosphatase is elevated while serum calcium and phosphorus levels are low. The metaphysis and epiphysis—the areas where growth is most active—are where the important radiographic features are seen, particularly at the distal ends of the radius, ulna, and femur as well as at the proximal ends of the tibia and fibula. Widening of the growth plate and cupping and flaring of the metaphysis, which appears disordered and "frayed," are indications of inadequate mineralisation in the provisional zone of calcification. Similar alterations are observed in the secondary ossification centres of the epiphysis; the bone turns radiolucent, loses sharpness at the perimeter, and bowing abnormalities usually occur (Figs. 15.1, 15.2, 15.3, 15.4 and 15.5).

Osteomalacia manifests after bone growth has stopped and is caused by the same pathomechanism as rickets; the word describes modifications to the axial and appendicular skeleton's cortical and trabecular bone. It is typically brought on by malabsorption syndrome, which leads to improper fat-soluble vitamin D absorption from the digestive tract. It might also be brought on by the proximal renal tubules malfunctioning, which would cause renal osteomalacia. This condition's most typical clinical manifestations are bone pain and muscular weakness. On radiographs, osteomalacia manifests as generalised osteopenia and many, bilateral, and frequently symmetric radiolucent lines, also known as pseudofractures or Looser zones, are observed in the cortex perpendicular to the long axis of the bone. These defects are widespread along the axillary margins of the scapulae, the inner margin of the femoral neck, the proximal dorsal aspect of the ulnae, the ribs, and the pubic and ischial rami. They are cortical insufficiency stress fractures filled with poorly mineralised callus, osteoid, and fibrous tissue.

Fig. 15.1 AP view of bilateral wrist joint showing osteopenia of the bones, widening of the growth plates of the distal radius and ulna, and flaring of the metaphyses

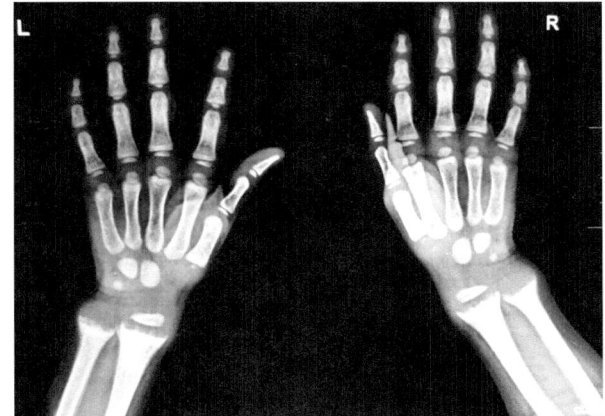

Fig. 15.2 AP view of bilateral knee joint showing widening, cupping, splaying, and fraying of physis of distal femur and proximal tibia

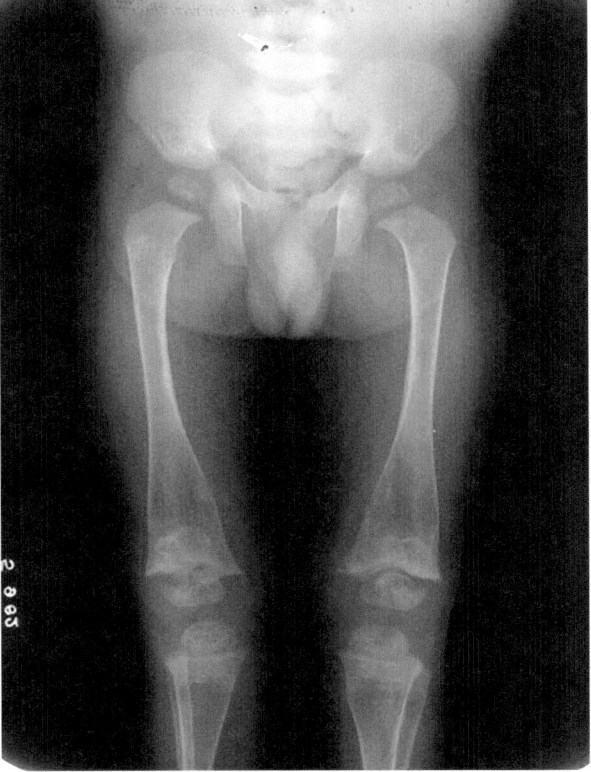

Fig. 15.3 AP view of bilateral wrist with forearm showing osteopenia of radius and ulna

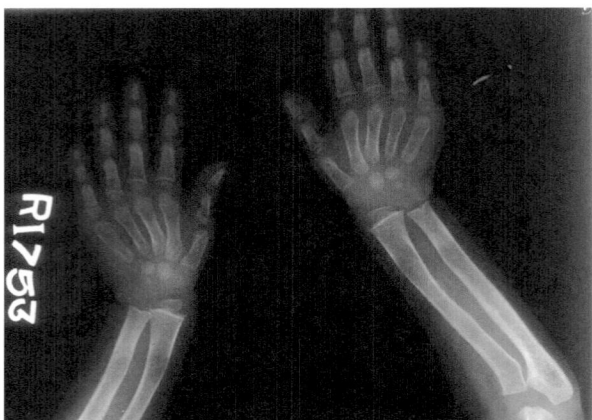

Fig. 15.4 AP view of bilateral wrist joint showing osteopenia of the bones, widening of the growth plates of the distal radius and ulna, and flaring of the metaphyses

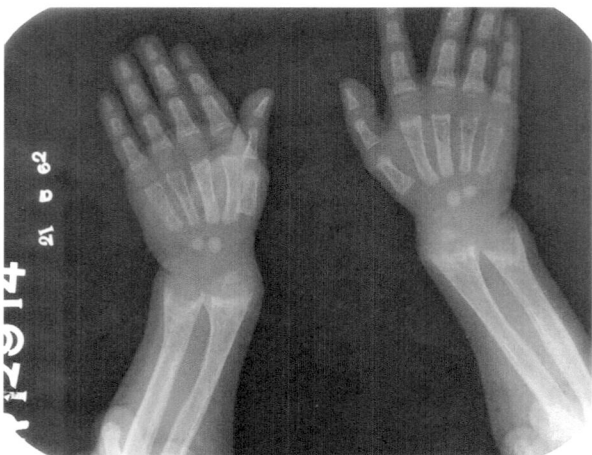

Fig. 15.5 AP view of pelvis showing generalised osteopenia with decreased mineralisation of femoral epiphysis due to rickets

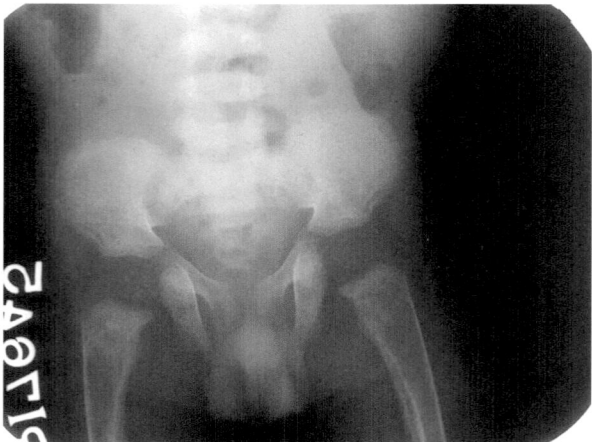

15.3   Hyperparathyroidism

The shoulder, hand, vertebrae, and skull are the primary target sites in the skeletal system for hyperparathyroidism. Its distinctive characteristics, including global osteopenia, subperiosteal, subchondral, and cortical bone resorption, brown tumours, and soft tissue and cartilage calcifications, may typically be seen with conventional radiography. On radiographs of the hands, subperiosteal resorption is particularly well visible. Although other bones can also be affected, it typically affects the radial portions of the middle phalanges of the middle and index fingers. Subchondral bone resorption is frequently present, leading to depression of the articular cartilage that lies above. Localised destructive changes in the bones caused by hyperparathyroidism manifest as brown tumours, which are a type of cyst-like lesion that can vary in size. These lesions can occur everywhere in the bones; however they typically occur in the jaw, pelvis, and femora (Figs. 15.6 and 15.7).

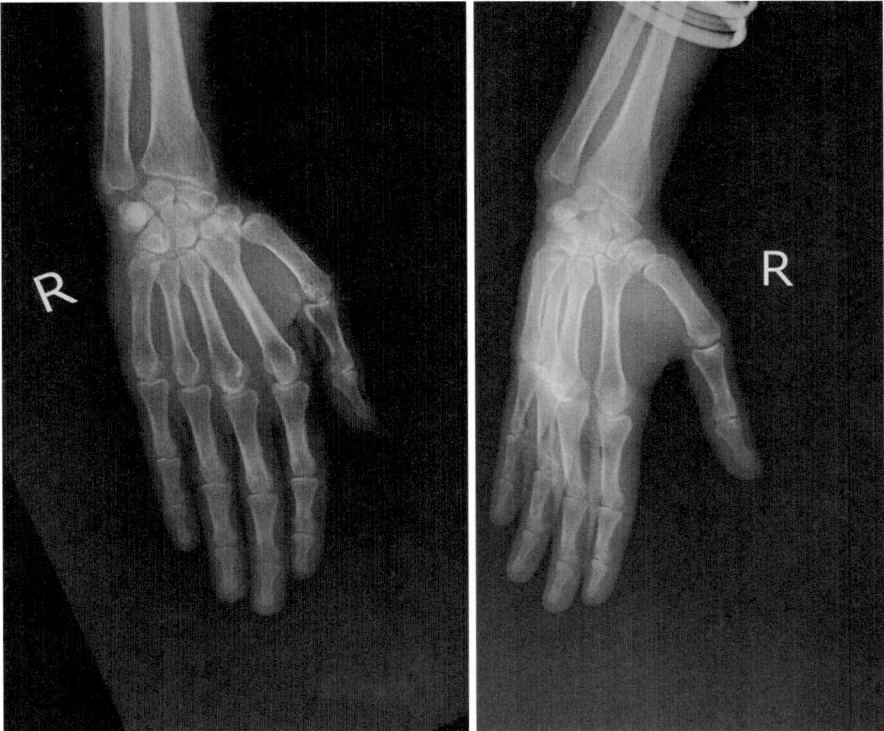

Fig. 15.6 X-ray of hand showing osteopenia of phalanges with subperiosteal resorption of bone in a case of hyperparathyroidism

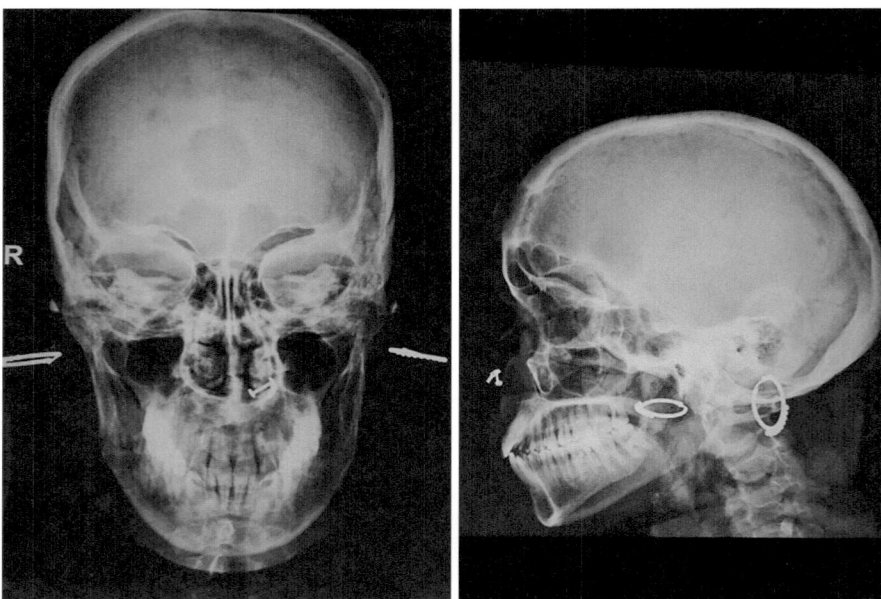

Fig. 15.7 X-ray of skull showing osteopenia with salt and pepper appearance in a case of hyperparathyroidism

Bibliography

1. Yochum TR, Rowe LJ. *Yochum and Rowe's Essentials of Skeletal Radiology.* 3rd ed. Philadelphia: Lippincott/Williams & Wilkins; 2005.
2. Greenspan A Beltran J. *Orthopedic Imaging: A Practical Approach.* Sixth ed. Philadelphia: Wolters Kluwer; 2015.

Part VII

Orthopaedic Surgical Procedures

Radiographs of Post-Surgical Orthopaedic Complications

Implant-related complications pose a significant concern in orthopaedic surgeries, and several common issues are associated with orthopaedic implants. These complications include:

Loosening: Over time, orthopaedic implants such as screws, plates, or artificial joints may become loose, resulting in pain, instability, and restricted mobility. Factors contributing to loosening include inadequate implant selection, poor bone quality, excessive stress on the implant, or infection. To address loosening, revision surgery may be required to replace or reposition the implant.

Infection: Implant-associated infections can occur following orthopaedic procedures, where bacteria colonise the implant surface, leading to persistent infection. Symptoms may include redness, swelling, warmth, increased pain, or discharge from the surgical site. Treating infection often involves implant removal and antibiotic treatment.

Fracture or Breakage: Orthopaedic implants used for fracture fixation or joint replacement can fracture or break under certain circumstances. Causes may include excessive stress, suboptimal implant design or quality, or traumatic events. In such cases, revision surgery is often necessary to remove the broken implant and replace it with a new one.

Malalignment or Malpositioning: Improper placement or positioning of orthopaedic implants can result in functional limitations, pain, and instability. These issues can arise due to surgical errors, technical challenges, or insufficient preoperative planning. Corrective surgery may be required to reposition the implant and restore optimal alignment and function.

Allergic Reactions: Although rare, some individuals may develop allergic reactions to certain implant materials, such as metal hypersensitivity. Allergic reactions can cause inflammation, pain, and tissue damage surrounding the implant. Treatment may involve switching to a different implant material or removing the implant to alleviate symptoms and prevent further complications.

N. S. Kushwaha, M. B. Abbas, *A Guide to Musculoskeletal Radiology*, https://doi.org/10.1007/978-981-99-6155-9_16

Wear and Tear: Implants, especially those used in joint replacements, can undergo wear and tear over time. This can lead to the release of particles or debris into the surrounding tissues, resulting in inflammation, pain, and potential implant failure. Regular monitoring, follow-up visits, and, if necessary, revision surgery may be necessary to address wear-related complications.

While implant-related complications are relatively rare, advancements in implant design, surgical techniques, and infection control have significantly reduced their occurrence. Orthopaedic surgeons closely monitor patients during follow-up visits and implement measures to minimise the risks associated with implants, ensuring optimal outcomes and long-term success of orthopaedic procedures (Figs. 16.1, 16.2, 16.3, 16.4, 16.5, 16.6, 16.7, 16.8, 16.9, 16.10, 16.11, 16.12, 16.13, 16.14 and 16.15).

Fig. 16.1 AP and lateral radiograph of humerus showing fracture shaft humerus managed by narrow dynamic compression plate with loosening of plate and screw with peri-implant osteolysis and nonunion

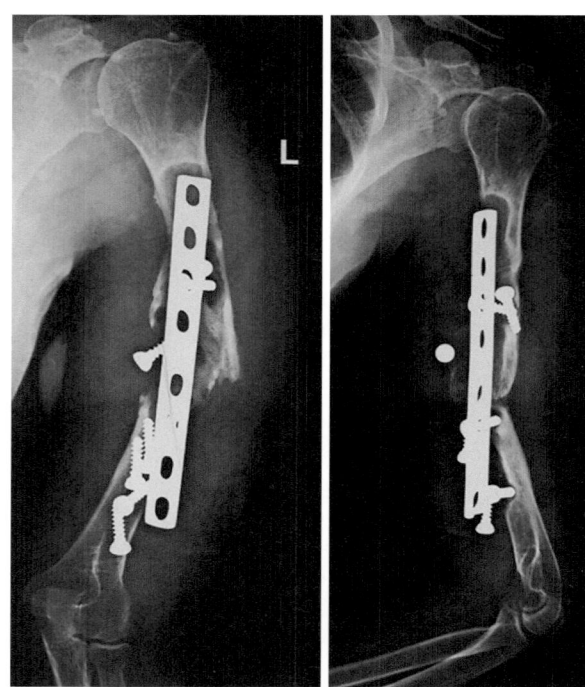

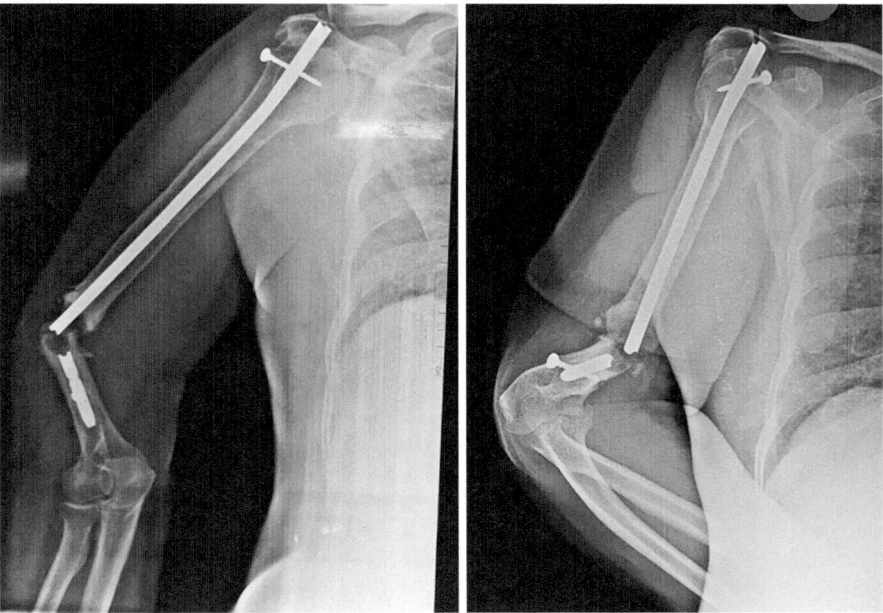

Fig. 16.2 AP and lateral radiograph of humerus showing fracture shaft humerus managed by humerus interlocking nail with broken humerus nail with nonunion of fracture in distal humerus

Fig. 16.3 AP and lateral radiograph of forearm showing united fracture both bone forearm fixed with small fragment dynamic compression plate with peri-implant fracture at the distal end of plate

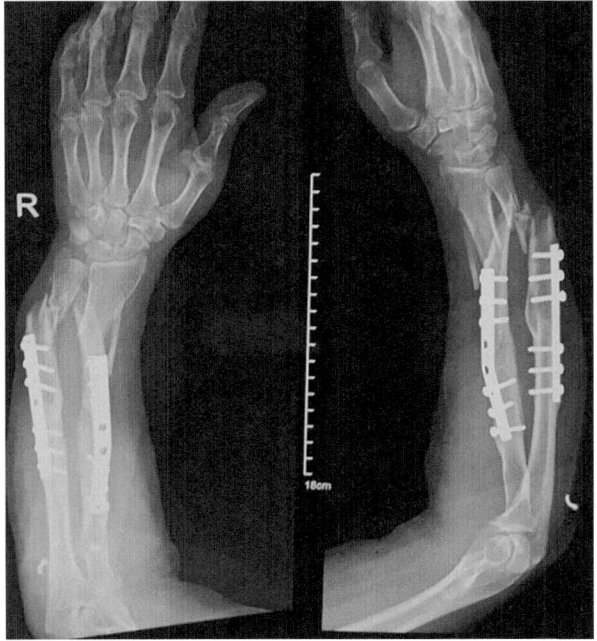

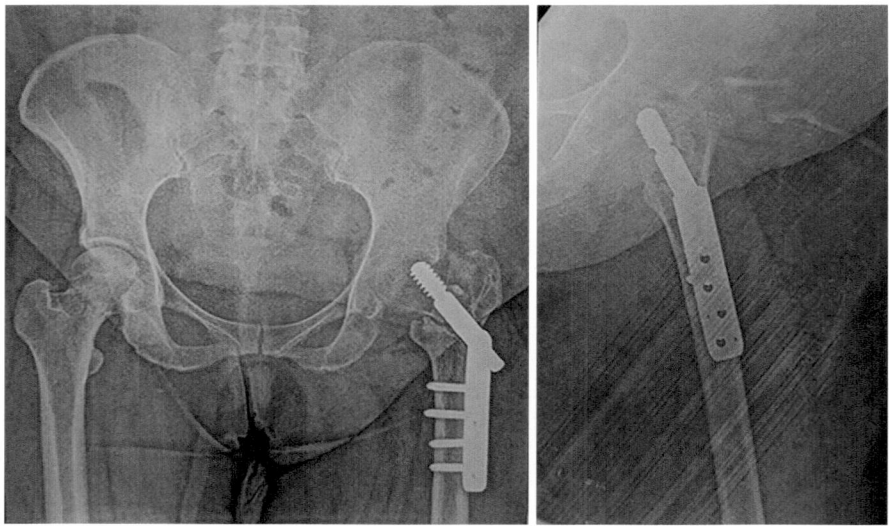

Fig. 16.4 X-ray pelvis with both hip showing fracture neck femur managed by DHS with screw cut out, varus collapse, nonunion, and AVN of head of femur

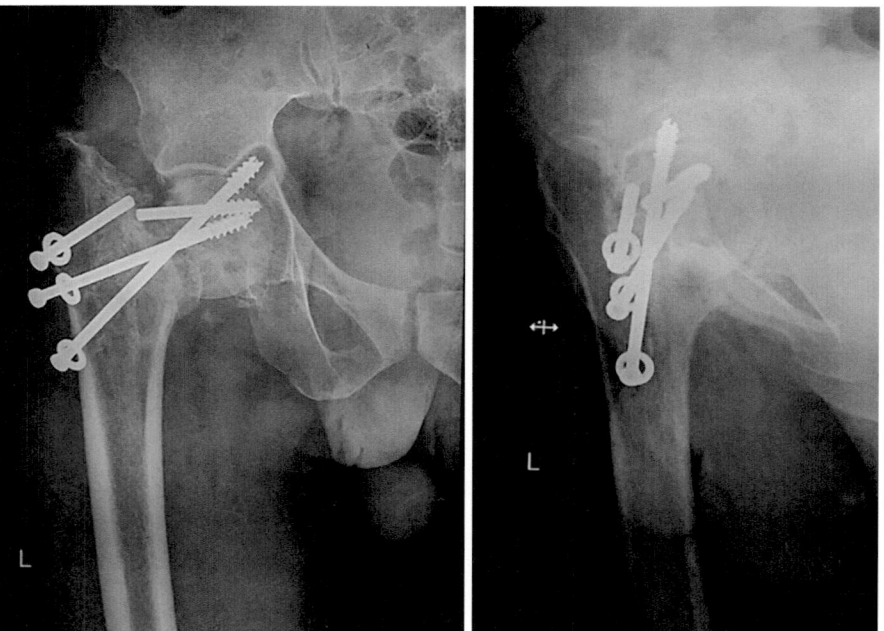

Fig. 16.5 X-ray showing fracture neck femur managed by cannulated cancellous screws with screw breakage and cut out with nonunion of the fracture

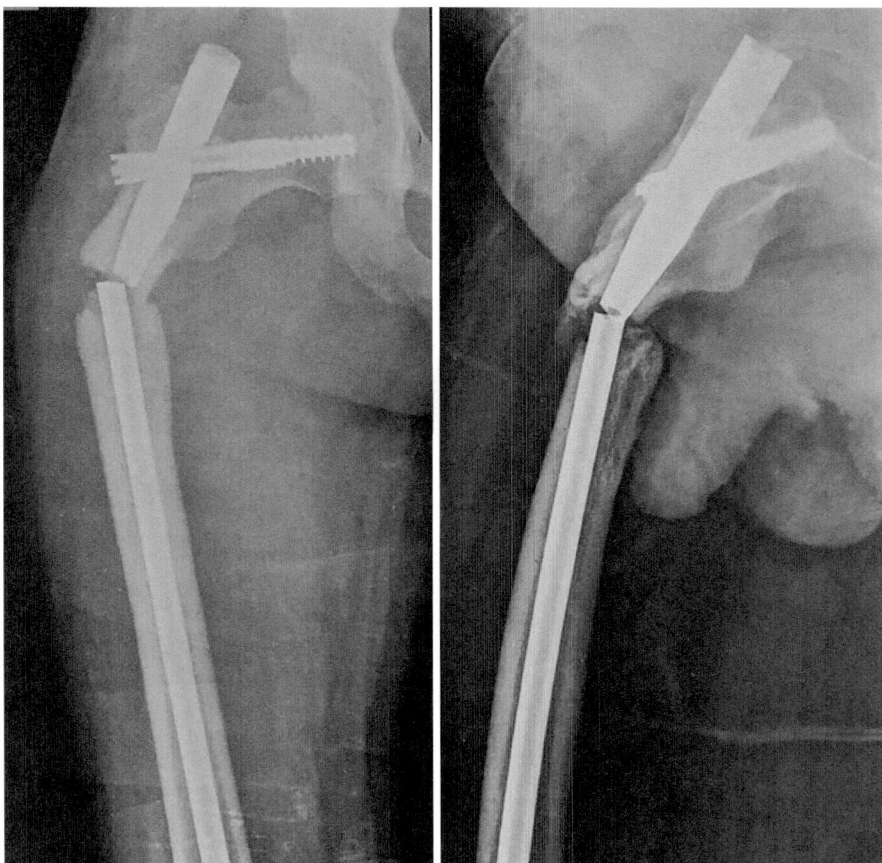

Fig. 16.6 X-ray showing subtrochanteric fracture managed by PFN with nonunion at the fracture site and implant breakage

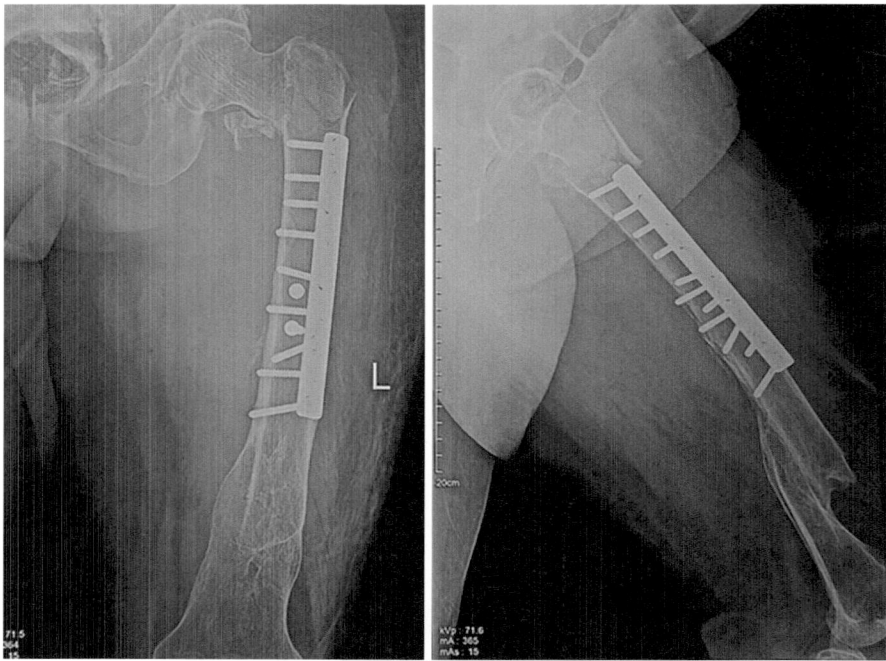

Fig. 16.7 X-ray showing united fracture shaft femur managed by broad DCP with peri-implant fracture at the proximal end

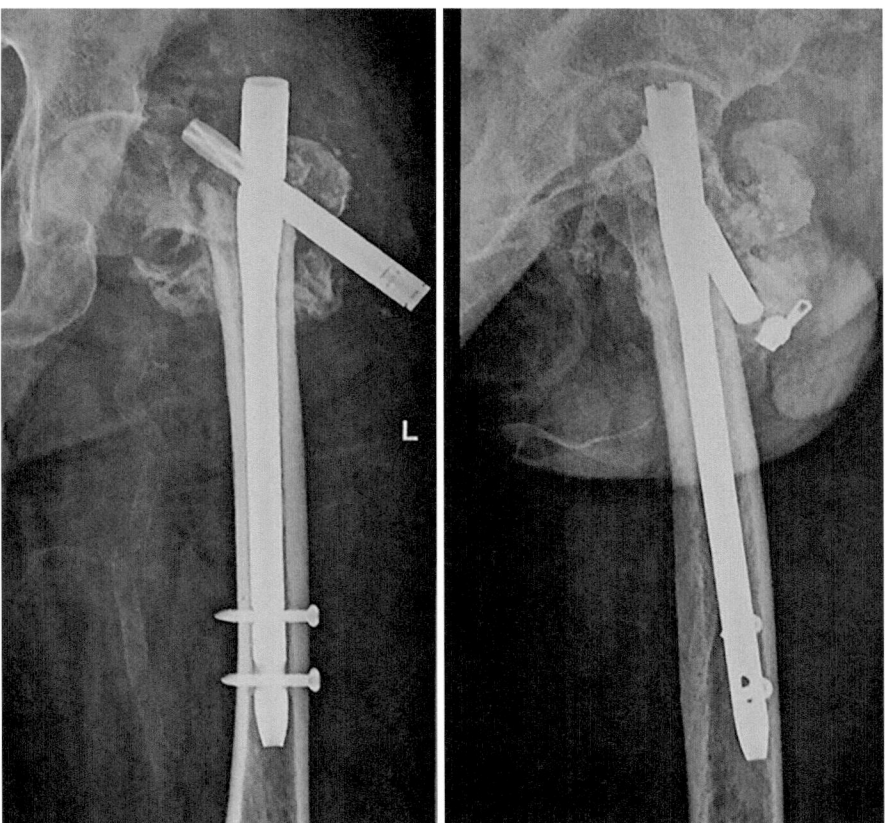

Fig. 16.8 X-ray showing intertrochanteric fracture managed by PFN with screw back out, varus collapse, and nonunion of fracture

Fig. 16.9 X-ray showing
united subtrochanteric
fracture managed by DCS
with peri-implant fracture
at the distal end

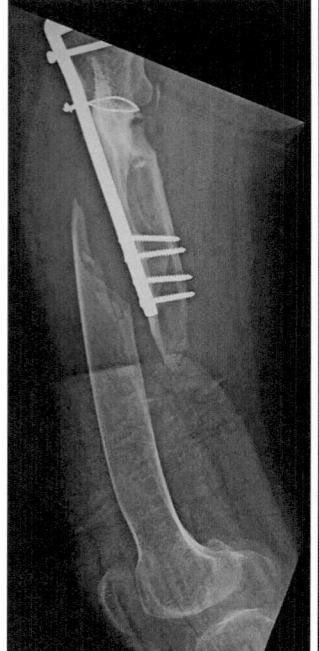
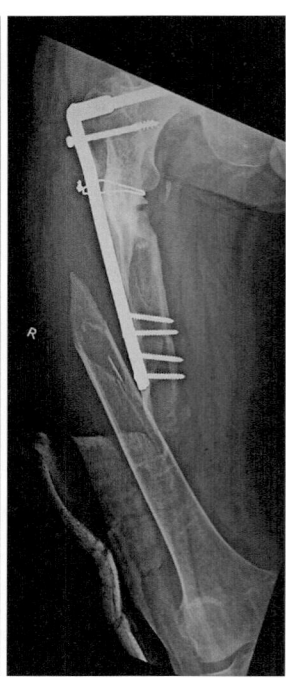

Fig. 16.10 X-ray showing
distal femur fracture
managed by distal femur
locking plate with
loosening of plate and
screws and nonunion of
fracture

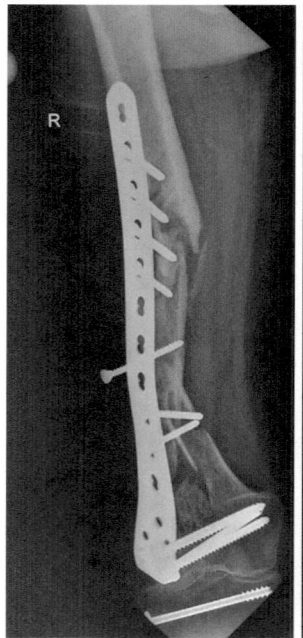
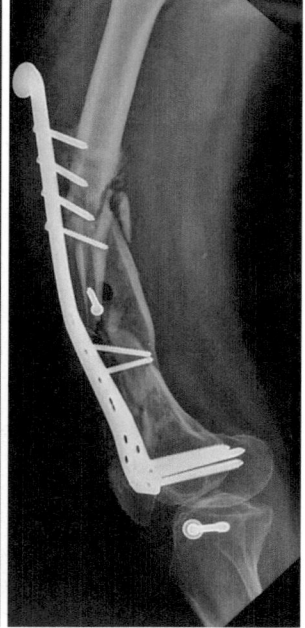

Fig. 16.11 X-ray showing fracture distal femur managed by dual plating with implant breakage and nonunion

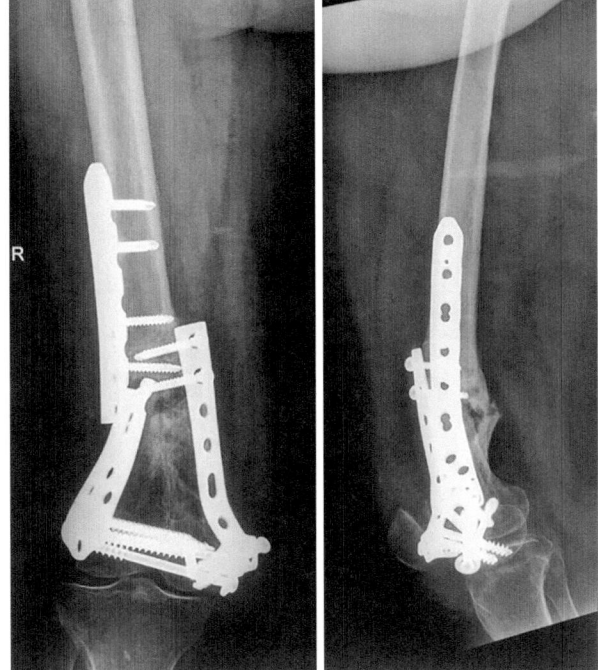

Fig. 16.12 X-ray showing bilateral hemiarthroplasty of the hip joint with protrusion-acetabuli due to acetabular wear

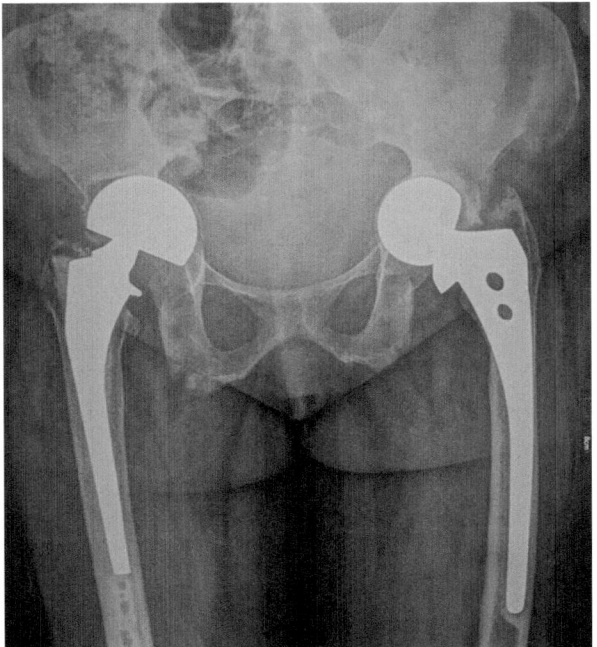

Fig. 16.13 X-ray showing hemiarthroplasty of right hip with aseptic osteolysis and implant loosening

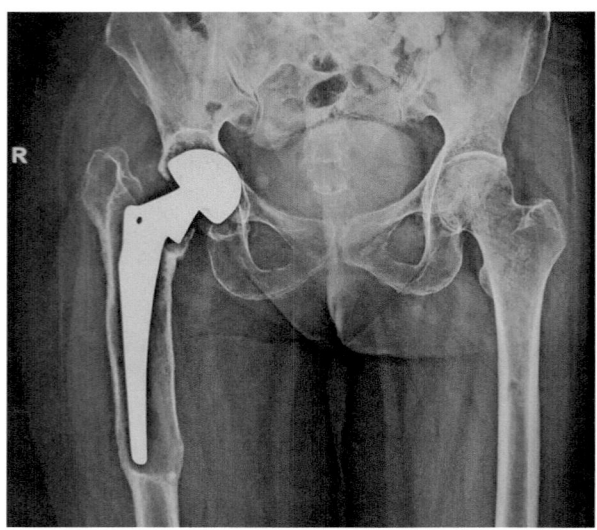

Fig. 16.14 X-ray showing peri-implant fracture in a patient with post cemented long stem THR

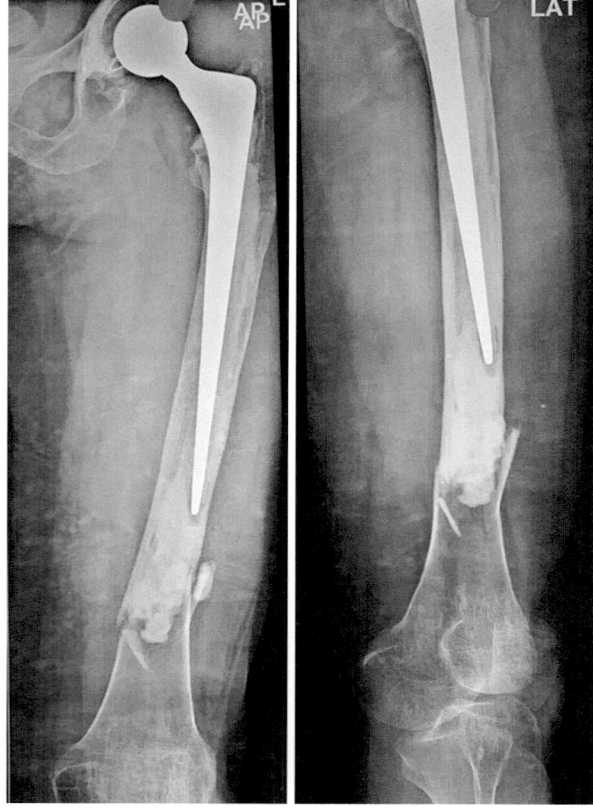

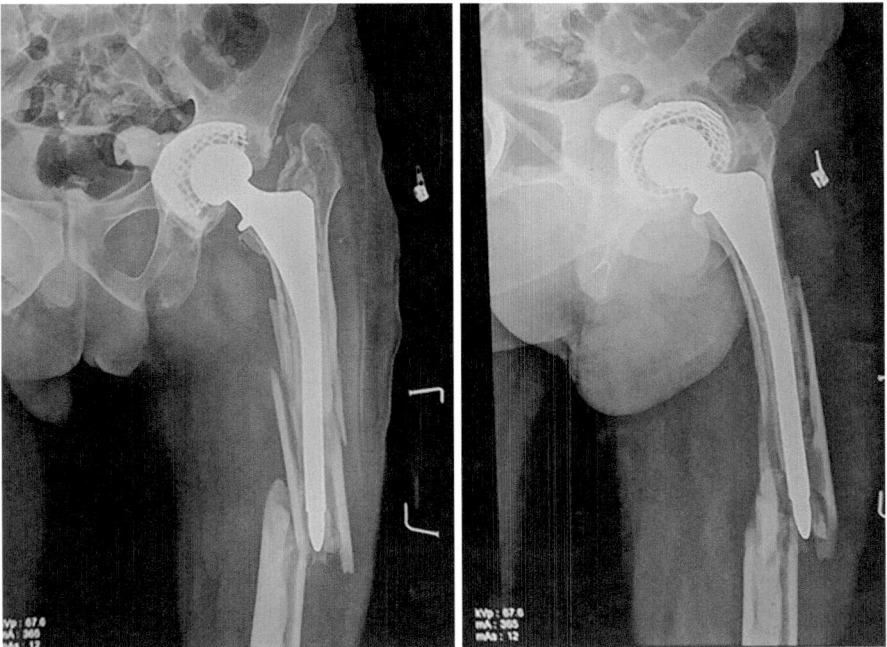

Fig. 16.15 X-ray showing peri-implant fracture in a post THR patient with stem loosening

Radiographs of Orthopaedic Reconstructive Procedures

17

Reconstructive procedures in orthopaedics encompass a wide range of interventions, including fracture fixation and joint replacement, which are vital for restoring functionality and improving the quality of life for individuals with musculoskeletal injuries or degenerative conditions. Fracture fixation aims to realign and stabilise broken bones, while joint replacement involves replacing damaged or arthritic joints with prosthetic implants. These procedures have revolutionised orthopaedic care, offering effective solutions to debilitating conditions and allowing patients to regain mobility, alleviate pain, and enhance their overall well-being.

Types of Implants for Fracture Fixation and Joint Replacement:

17.1 Fracture Fixation Implants

Screws: Various types and sizes of screws, such as cortical and cancellous screws, are used to hold fractured bone fragments together during the healing process.

Plates: Rigid metal plates, secured with screws, are utilised to stabilise and support fractured bones, particularly in cases of complex fractures or those involving bones near joints.

Intramedullary Nails: These implants are inserted into the intramedullary canal of long bones, providing stability and support while allowing weight-bearing during the healing process.

External Fixators: Pins or wires are inserted into the bone on either side of the fracture and connected to an external frame to hold the fractured bones in proper alignment.

17.2   Joint Replacement Implants

Total Joint Replacement: Damaged or arthritic joints are completely replaced with prosthetic implants, typically made of metal (titanium or cobalt-chromium alloys) and featuring bearing surfaces made of materials like polyethylene or ceramic. Total joint replacement is commonly performed in hip, knee, shoulder, and elbow joints.

Partial Joint Replacement: Only the damaged portion of the joint is replaced with a prosthetic implant, preserving the healthy parts of the joint. Examples include unicompartmental knee replacement and hemiarthroplasty for the hip.

Reverse Joint Replacement: This procedure is utilised in specific cases of shoulder arthritis, where the normal joint anatomy is reversed. The ball component is fixed to the shoulder blade (scapula), and the socket component is attached to the upper arm bone (humerus), providing stability and improved function.

Resurfacing Joint Replacement: In hip resurfacing, the surface of the joint is capped with a metal implant, preserving the femoral head while replacing the damaged joint surfaces, allowing for improved joint function.

It is important to note that the choice of implant depends on factors such as the type and location of the fracture or joint condition, the patient's anatomy, and the surgeon's expertise. Orthopaedic surgeons carefully select the appropriate implants for each individual case, aiming to achieve optimal stability, functionality, and long-term success in fracture fixation and joint replacement procedures (Figs. 17.1, 17.2, 17.3, 17.4, 17.5, 17.6, 17.7, 17.8, 17.9, 17.10, 17.11, 17.12, 17.13, 17.14, 17.15 and 17.16).

Fig. 17.1 AP and lateral view of arm showing fracture mid-shaft of humerus fixed with open reduction internal fixation with dynamic compression plating

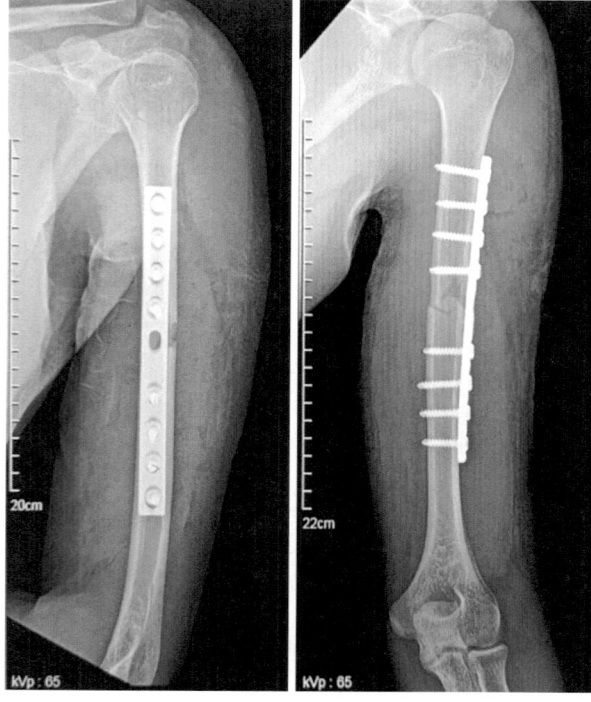

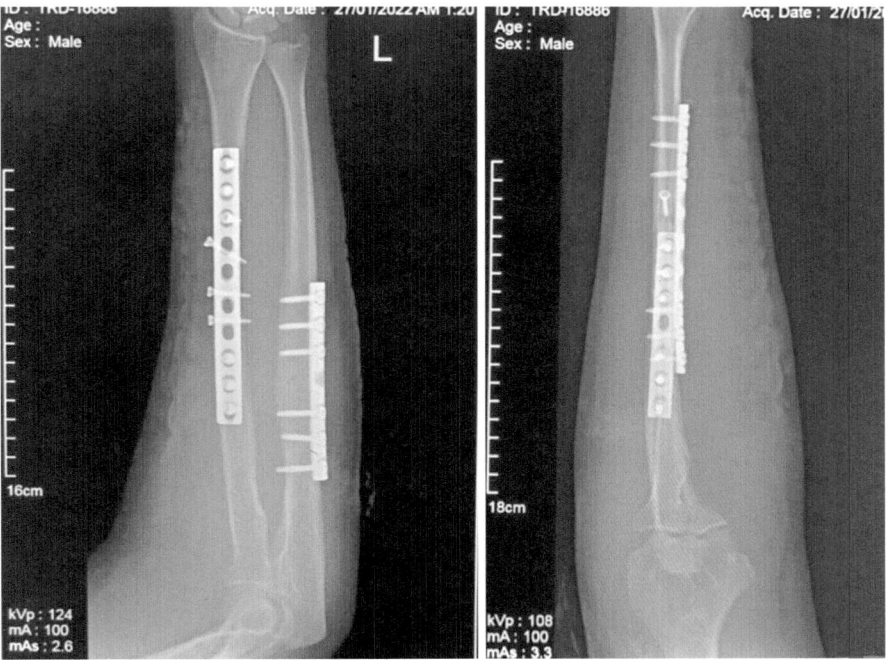

Fig. 17.2 AP and lateral view of forearm showing fracture shaft of radius and ulna fixed with open reduction and internal fixation with dynamic compression plating

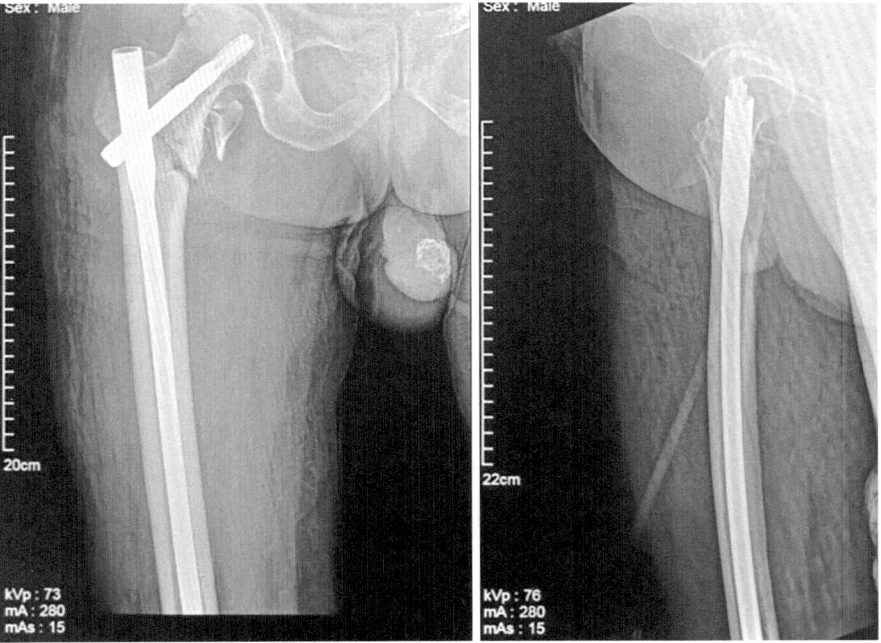

Fig. 17.3 AP and lateral view of hip showing intertrochanteric fracture fixed with closed reduction and internal fixation with proximal femoral nail antirotation

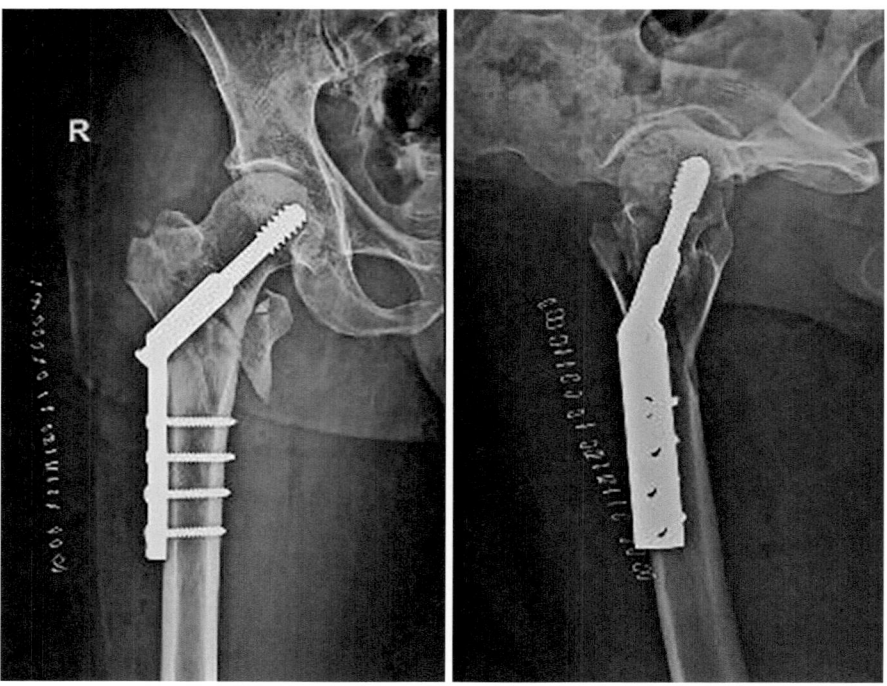

Fig. 17.4 AP and lateral view of hip showing intertrochanteric fracture fixed by open reduction internal fixation with dynamic hip screw

Fig. 17.5 AP view of pelvis showing acetabular fracture of the posterior wall and column fixed with open reduction and internal fixation with recon plate and screws

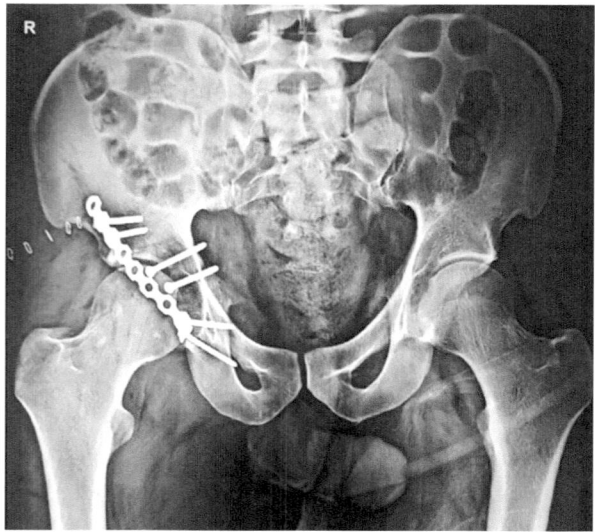

Fig. 17.6 AP view of
pelvis showing total hip
replacement done in a
patient with post-traumatic
arthritis of hip due to
acetabular fracture

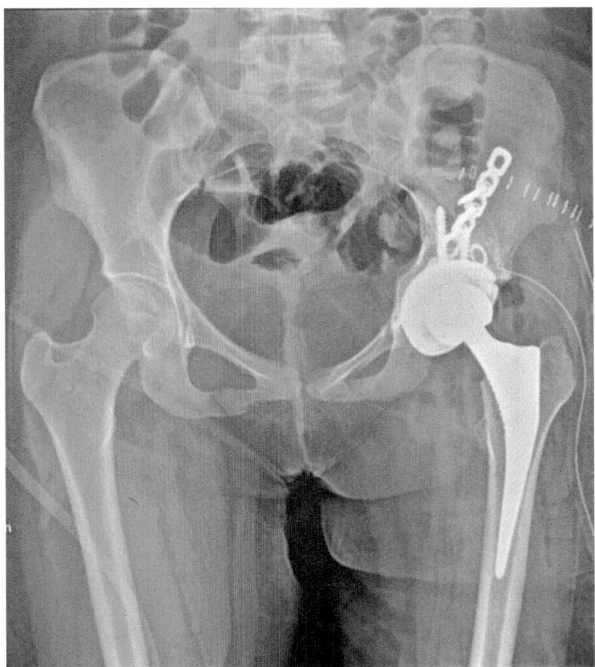

Fig. 17.7 AP view of
pelvis showing
hemiarthroplasty done with
modular bipolar prosthesis
in a geriatric patient with
fracture neck of femur

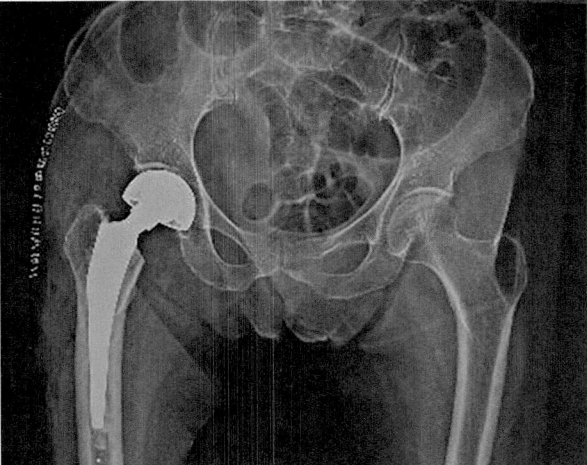

Fig. 17.8 AP and lateral view of leg showing fracture proximal shaft tibia fixed with closed reduction and internal fixation with tibial interlocking nail

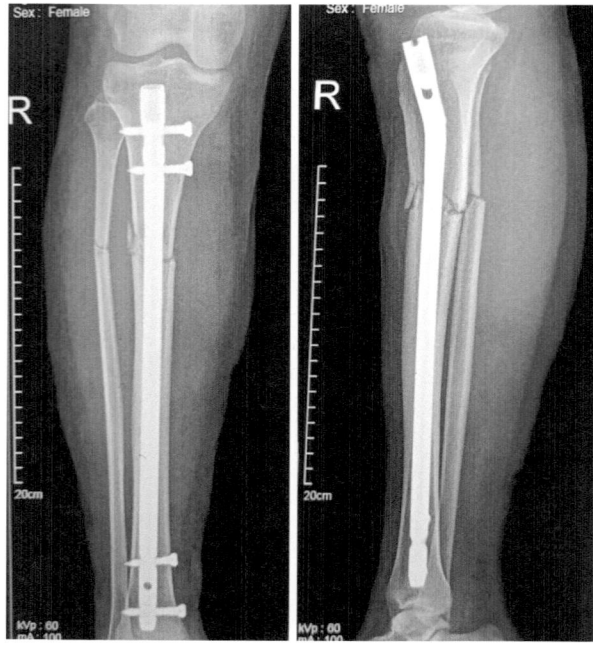

Fig. 17.9 AP and lateral view of knee showing megaprosthesis of knee joint done in a patient with giant cell tumour of distal femur

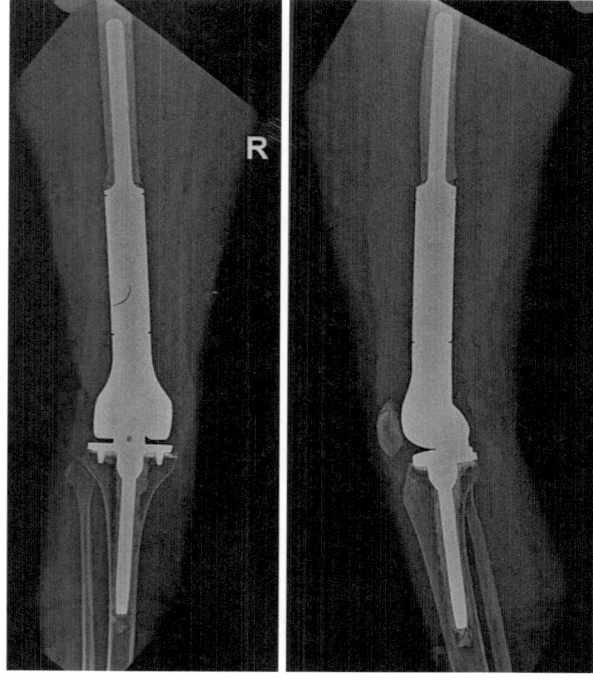

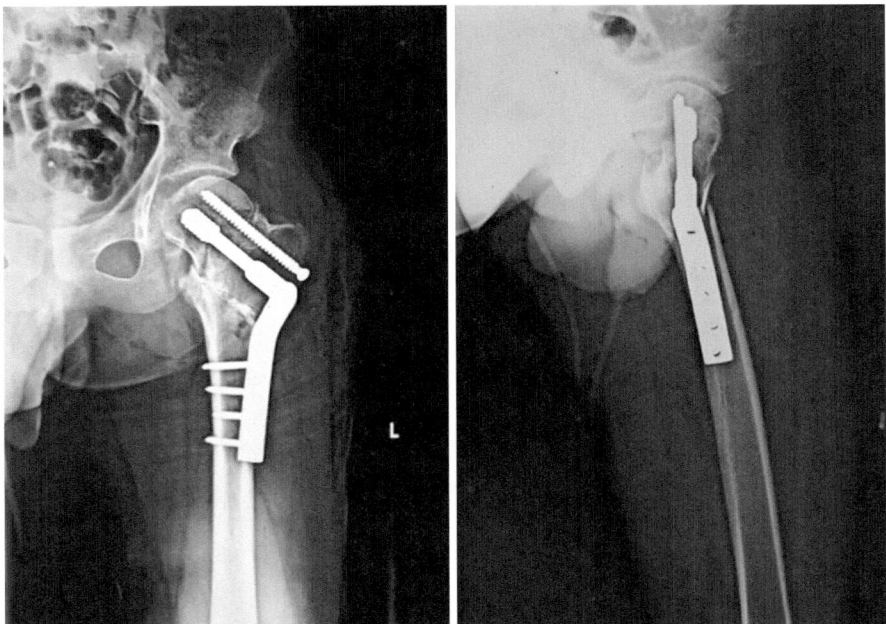

Fig. 17.10 AP and lateral view of hip showing nonunion fracture neck femur in young male fixed with closed reduction internal fixation with valgus osteotomy with double angled dynamic hip screw

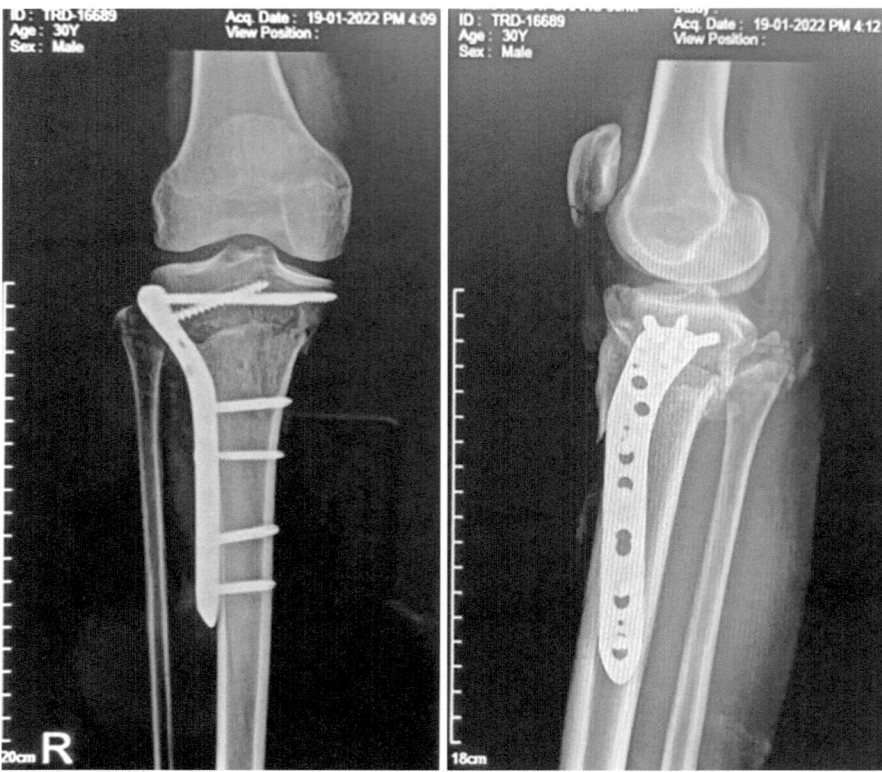

Fig. 17.11 AP and lateral view of knee with proximal leg showing fracture proximal tibia fixed with open reduction internal fixation with proximal tibial locking plate

Fig. 17.12 AP and lateral view of distal femur with knee showing intercondylar fracture of distal femur fixed by open reduction internal fixation with distal femur locked plate and a medial T plate

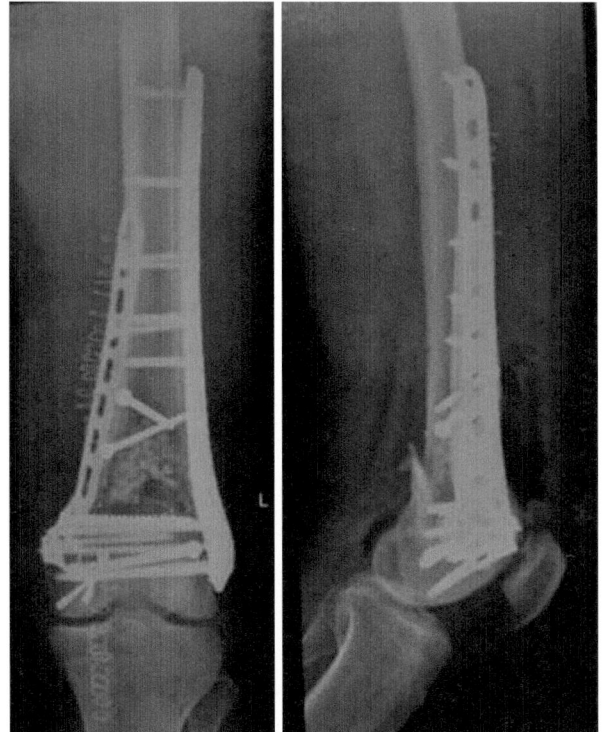

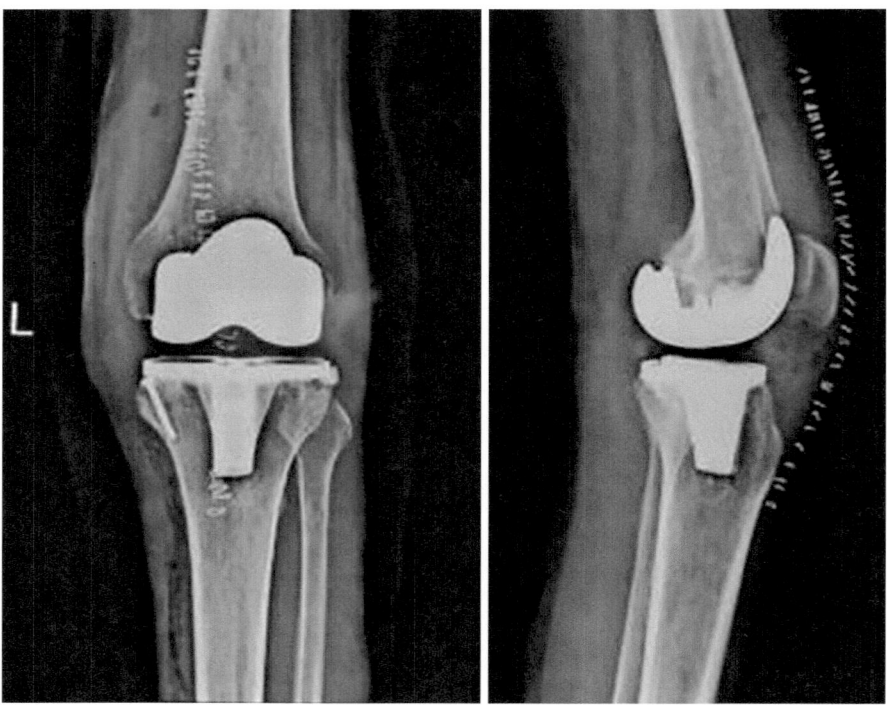

Fig. 17.13 AP and lateral view of knee joint showing total knee replacement done in a patient with osteoarthritis of the knee

Fig. 17.14 AP and lateral view of the knee showing transverse fracture of patella fixed by open reduction internal fixation with tension band wiring

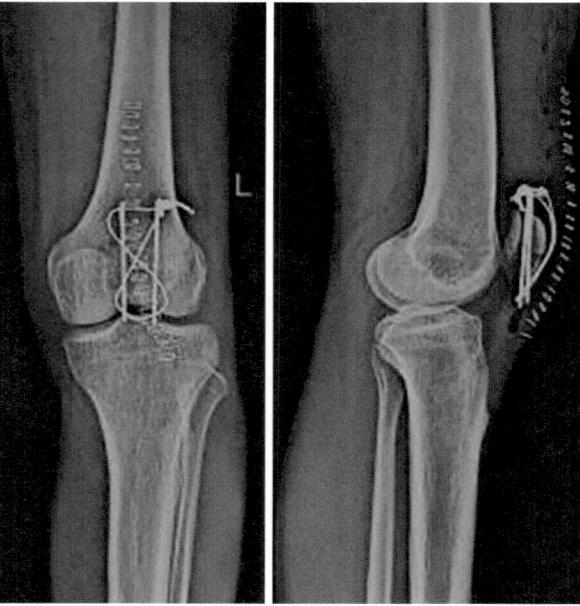

Fig. 17.15 AP and lateral view of dorso-lumbar spine showing fracture L1 vertebrae fixed by open reduction and posterior stabilisation with pedicle screw and rod system with decompression of spinal cord

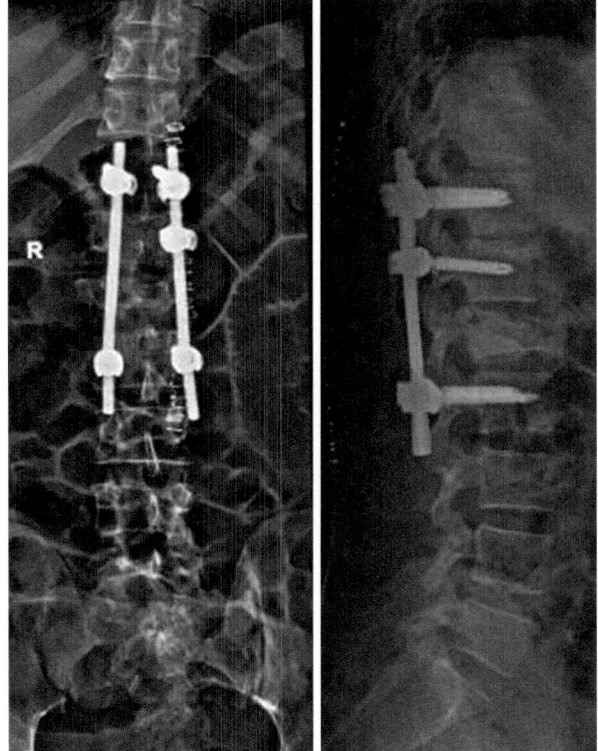

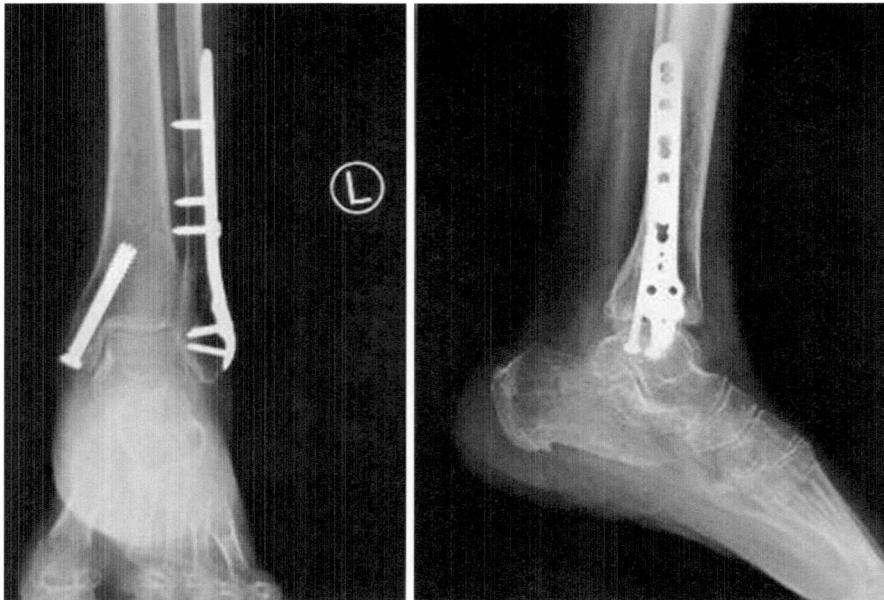

Fig. 17.16 AP and lateral view of ankle joint showing united bimalleolar fracture fixed by open reduction internal fixation of medial malleolus by cannulated cancellous screws and open reduction internal fixation of lateral malleolus by distal fibular locked plate